MOUNT MARY COLLEGE LIBRARY
Milwaukee, Wisconsin 53222
WITHDRAWN

W9-BWD-325

What is the limbic system?
How do nerves transmit messages?
How do we cope with 'jet lag'?
What happens when we suffer a stroke?
What is the significance of dreaming?
How does a child learn to speak?
Is senile deterioration a reality?
How do we perceive the outside world?
What do electroencephalograms tell us?
Which side of the brain is logical, and which artistic?
How does the brain sort and store its information?
Can the brain be fooled?
What is extrasensory perception?
How are our bodily functions monitored and controlled?
How does the brain cope with physical damage or drug abuse?
What are reflexes?
How well do we understand the troubled mind?
Where are the centers of speech, hunger, and emotion?
How does man's brain differ from those of other mammals?
How can we measure intelligence – or creativity?
Are sex and sexuality the same thing?

The Brain
A User's Manual

These and countless other questions are answered here in words and pictures that can be understood by everyone – providing a complete layman's guide to the innermost workings of the body's most complex and remarkable organ.

THE DIAGRAM GROUP has achieved world-wide recognition as the creator of this unique format for presenting the most up-to-date medical knowledge simply, clearly, and immediately. Previous books by the group, including **Man's Body, Woman's Body, Child's Body, The Healthy Body,** and **Sex: A User's Manual,** have been published in 17 languages throughout the world and have sold more than 5 million copies in 20 countries.

MOUNT MARY COLLEGE LIBRARY
Milwaukee, Wisconsin 53222
WITHDRAWN

The. Brain

A User's Manual

The Diagram Group

A Perigee Book

83-1716

Perigee Books
are published by
G. P. Putnam's Sons
200 Madison Avenue
New York, New York 10016

Copyright © 1982 by Diagram Visual Information
Limited. All rights reserved. This book, or parts
thereof, may not be reproduced in any form
without permission.

Library of Congress Cataloging in Publication Data
Main entry under title:

The Brain.

  "A Perigee book."
  Bibliography: p.
  Includes index.
  1. Brain.   I. Diagram Group.
QP376.B6958 1982b   612'.82   81-17942
ISBN 0-399-50622-5   AACR2

First Perigee printing, 1982

Printed in the United States of America

612.82
B73

The Diagram Group

Editors	David Lambert Martyn Bramwell Gail Lawther	Art Editors	Mark Evans Richard Hummerstone Kathleen McDougall
Contributors	Ruth Swann Susan Bosanko Roger Cohen Ruth Midgley Katherine M. Seed	Artists	Sean Gilbert Brian Hewson Janos Marffy Graham Rosewarne
Researchers	Enid Moore Elizabeth Pring	Assistant artists	Neil Copleston Ashley Haddock Debra Lee Steve Levington Joseph Robinson Max Rutherford
Indexer	Mary Ling		

Editorial Consultants

Dr. C.M.C. Allen M.A., M.B., B.B.Chir., M.R.C.P.
Hon. Lecturer in Neurology
Guy's Hospital, London

Dr. J.N. Blau M.D., F.R.C.P., F.R.C.Path.
Consultant Neurologist
The National Hospitals for Nervous Diseases, London,
and Northwick Park Hospital, London

Dr. Gwyneth Lewis M.B.B.S., M.R.C.G.P.
Medical Officer
The University of Sussex

Dr. Colette Ray
Lecturer in Psychology
Brunel University, Uxbridge

Mr. P.L. Richardson M.B., Ch.B.(Edin.), F.R.C.S.(Eng.)
Senior Neurosurgical Registrar
Maudsley Hospital, London

Dr. M.K. Thompson M.B., Ch.B., F.R.C.G.P.
General Practitioner
Croydon, Surrey

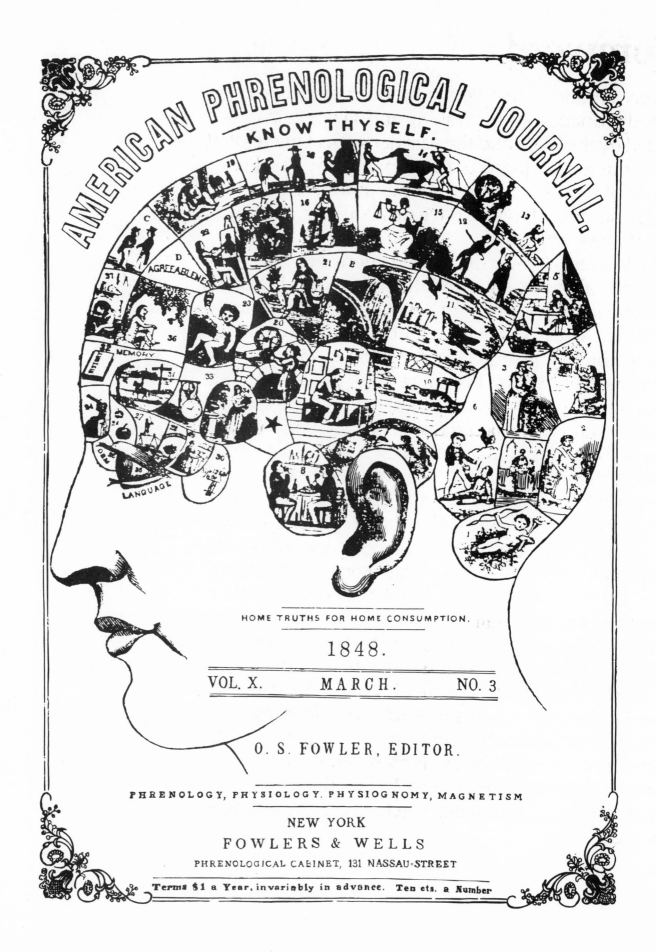

AMERICAN PHRENOLOGICAL JOURNAL.

KNOW THYSELF.

HOME TRUTHS FOR HOME CONSUMPTION.

1848.

VOL. X.   MARCH.   NO. 3

O. S. FOWLER, EDITOR.

PHRENOLOGY, PHYSIOLOGY, PHYSIOGNOMY, MAGNETISM

NEW YORK

FOWLERS & WELLS

PHRENOLOGICAL CABINET, 131 NASSAU-STREET

Terms $1 a Year, invariably in advance.   Ten cts. a Number

Foreword

Every emotion, every thought, every dream, act, and bodily function of our waking and sleeping lives is ruled by the brain and the vast network of nerves that fans out to every part of the human body. And yet most of us know more about our automobiles and domestic plumbing than we do about the way we think, feel, and act.

The last few decades have seen enormous advances in medical knowledge, and the editors of THE BRAIN believe it is time for the mystery and confusion to be stripped away. We believe that by understanding the brain and its functions, its strengths and its weaknesses, we can live more fully, understand our own abilities and behavior (and that of others) more readily, and make better use of our own physical, mental and emotional potential.

Our goal in this book has been to present this remarkable organ in terms the general reader can understand easily and immediately. Simple, clear anatomical drawings plot the innermost parts of the brain and describe their key functions, while charts and diagrams display medical statistics in a way that is comprehensible to all.

During the creation of this book, text and illustrations were submitted to a team of medical advisors for careful checking and approval. Their authority, and the DIAGRAM visual approach, will, we hope, provide an invaluable family reference guide and a source of information, enjoyment, and understanding of the human brain – the most complex and astonishing 'mechanism' in the natural world.

Contents

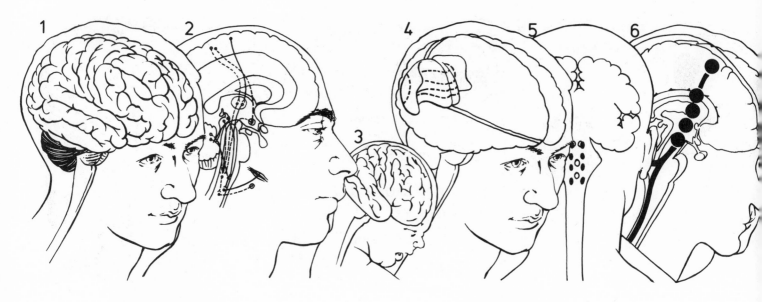

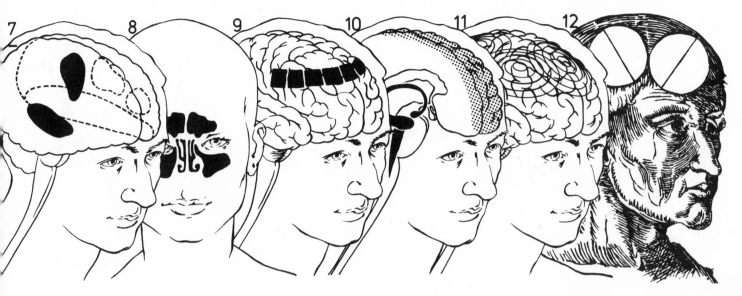

Chapter 1

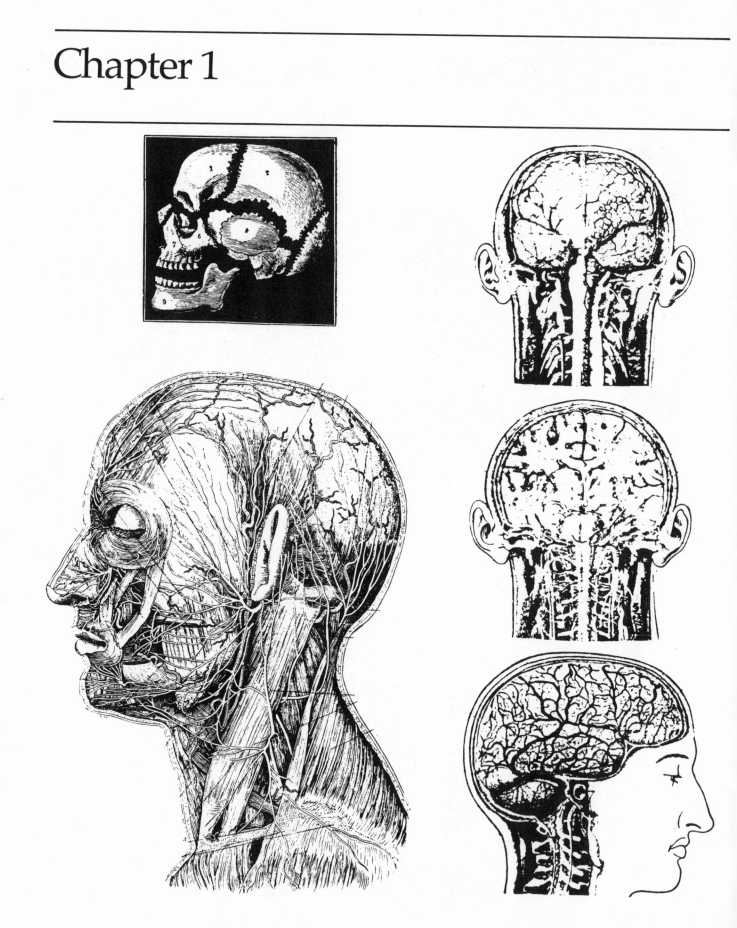

ANATOMY OF THE BRAIN

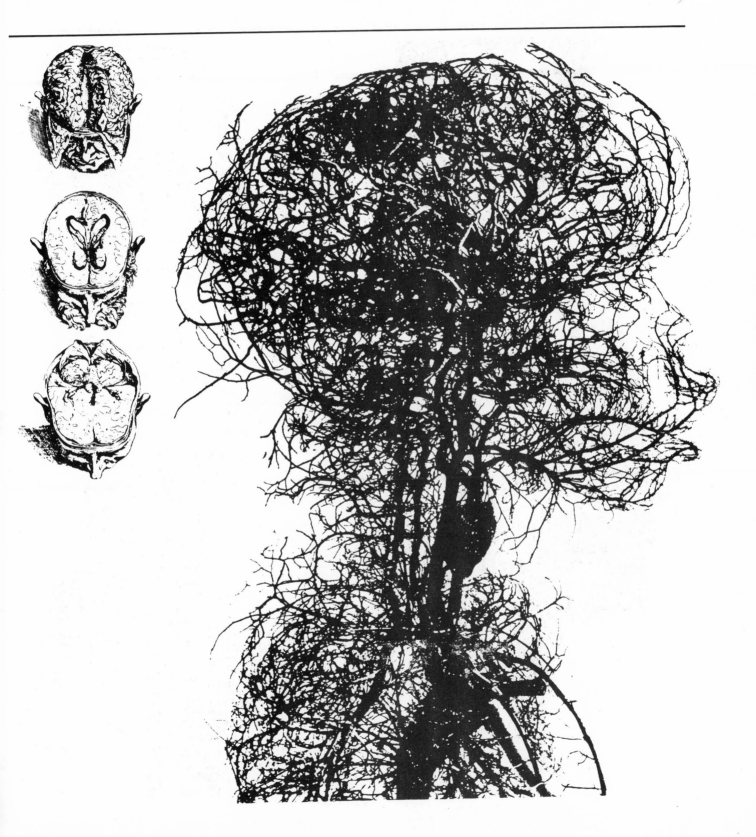

The Brain

For 40,000 years, people mentally as well equipped as you or I unknowingly carried in their skulls the source of their emotions – an amazing organ that was also to devise farming, invent the wheel, subdue disease, send men into space, and make us masters of more than a million other kinds of living thing that share our world.

Maybe it is not really surprising that thinking people failed to recognize the brain for what it was. After all, the brain is nothing much to look at – just an outsize "walnut" with the consistency of soft, moist, cheese. Understandably, the ancient Greek philosopher Aristotle credited the heart with thinking and sensing, and gave the brain the servile task of cooling blood.

Much about the brain remains a puzzle. But scientific studies – several acclaimed in the Nobel Prize awards of 1981 – have shown beyond all doubt the human brain to be the most amazing mechanism on our planet. Packed into this lump little bigger than a grapefruit are billions of cells. If each were a grain of sand, the lot would fill a truck. Only 10 billion – one-tenth of the total – are evidently active nerve cells. But each of these has actual or potential links with tens of thousands of others. Thanks to chemical messengers, electric impulses constantly flash into, through and from the brain. Inside, special regions sift, reject or pass on to others a host of freshly sensed experiences, matching these with ones already memorized. By such means the brain shapes and directs our conscious and unconscious feelings, thoughts and actions.

Compared with a big up-to-date computer the human brain seems slow and ineffectual. Computers can outcalculate us any day.

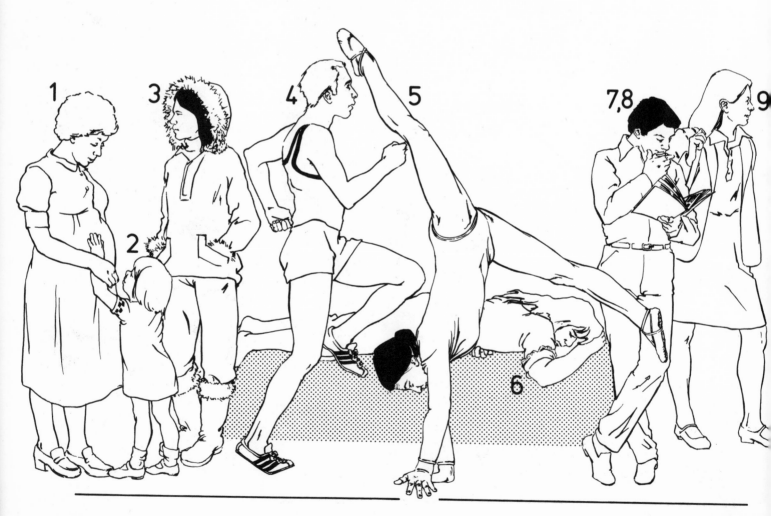

Computer-operated robots can build automobiles – even robots – with inhuman speed and accuracy. Yet no computer can make a robot walk, run, swim, climb, drive, tie a knot, write, speak, memorize a route, plan a shopping list, hate and fall in love. Its ability to manipulate your body in so many ways and situations is what makes the brain such an astonishing creation.

That structure took hundreds of millions of years to forge, and the brain's convolutions bear traces of its evolutionary past. What at first looks like a simple corrugated lump is a complex organ built up of different parts – some large, some small – rather like a shack that has been enlarged bit by bit into a mansion. Let's start by glancing at the brain in its entirety before we peek into the rooms inside.

Brain Power
The figures below remind us of the many ways in which our brains determine and control the workings of our bodies.
1 Affection.
2 Growth.
3 Body temperature control.
4 Coordinated movement.
5 Balance.
6 Sleep.
7 Learning.
8 Taste.
9 Speech.
10 Moral judgment.
11 Problem solving.
12 Hand-eye coordination.
13 Aggression.
14 Creativity.
15 Meditation.
16 Sexuality.

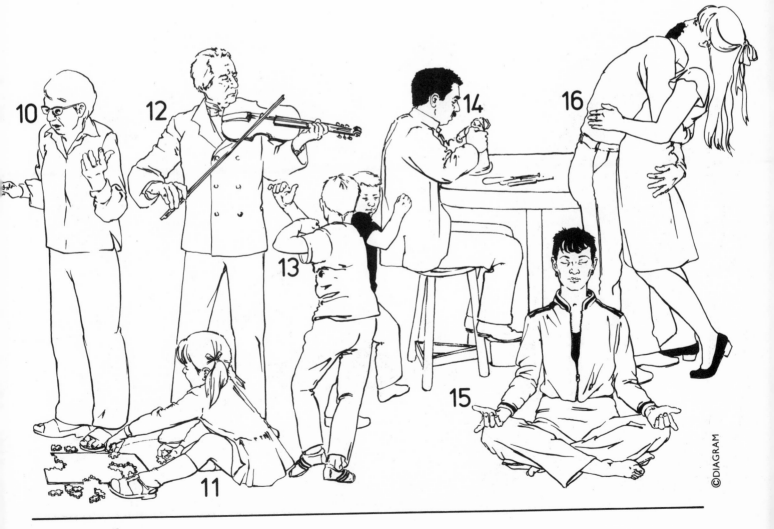

©DIAGRAM

Brain Size

Many people assume that man owes his intelligence entirely to his brain's large size. These two pages help to show how far that popular belief is justified.

No one questions that man's brain is big. Our lifesize illustration of a brain seen from above shows just how large it is. The brain of an average white adult male tips the scales at about 3lb (1.4kg), or half the weight of a newborn human baby. Reckoned by capacity, the same brain fills some 85 cubic inches (1400cc), or the space taken by 3 US pints of milk.

But brain size varies both between sexes and among the world's races. Women, for example, tend to have smaller brains than men, which is not surprising as women also tend to have smaller bodies than men. If brain size directly related to

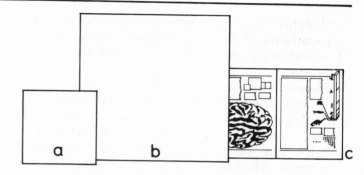

Surface area
Shown (below) is a human brain drawn lifesize from above. In fact this gives a misleading idea of the brain's surface area. Only one-third of that surface is normally on view. The remainder lies hidden by the folds. The diagram (above) compares the area of the normally visible surface (**a**) with the total surface area if spread flat to its full 324sq.in. (**b**) – both shown to a common scale with two pages of this book (**c**).

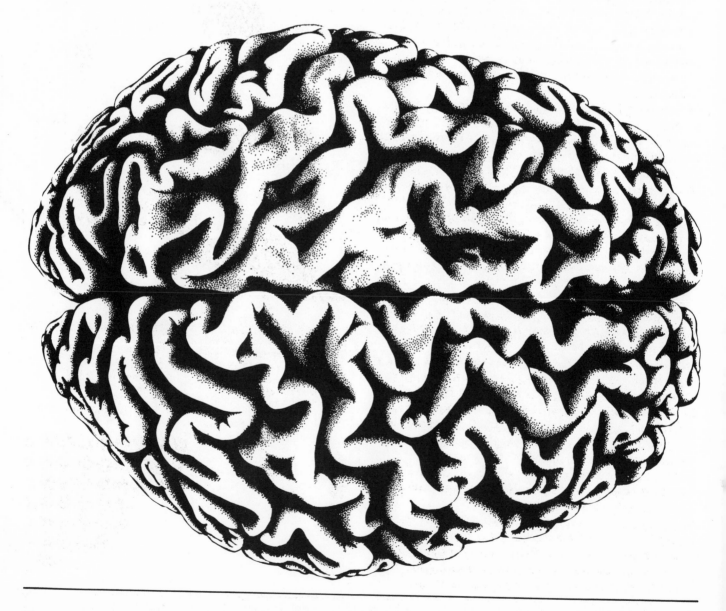

intelligence, then the big-brained Eskimos might well outthink all other racial groups. However, even within the same sex or race we find great variations.

But research suggests such differences can be misleading. For instance, someone with a brain no more than two-thirds normal size may be of average or even greater intelligence. The French novelist Anatole France (1844–1924) had just such a tiny brain. On the other hand, one of the largest brains ever measured was an idiot's. Studies of bright, dim and average individuals have failed to link brain size to intellectual capacity. So brain size taken on its own seems a poor guide to intelligence.

Brain size in relation to body size, however, is more meaningful. Scientists find that tall people have heavier brains than short ones, but that in relation to their height, the short people have bigger brains and heads than the tall ones and are at least as intelligent. Brain surface area provides what may be an even more telling comparison between individuals.

Matching relative brain size to intelligence shows up some sharp differences between man and other animals. We find, for example, that a man's brain is more than three times heavier than a gorilla's, although that great ape weighs three times more than a man. Moving away from our hominoid kin we discover even more discrepancy. A horse ten times heavier than a man has a brain less than half the weight of his. An elephant's brain admittedly outweighs a man's by three and a half times, but the difference between their overall body weights is much greater than that.

Even brain/body ratio gives only a rough guide to intelligence. Bulk for bulk, house mice, porpoises, squirrel monkeys and tree shrews all have more impressive brain/body ratios than we do. Yet, plainly, these beasts – porpoises perhaps excepted – are intellectual pygmies compared with people. What makes us mentally so different from them is less how much brain we store in our skulls than what kind of brain this is. The immense superiority of your brain over a beast's lies in your brain's greater internal complexity – the organization betrayed by its big, deeply wrinkled cerebral hemispheres, giving a huge surface area to the part that really does the thinking.

In every individual, however, cerebral and indeed overall brain size does not remain constant through life. Brain weight increases more than three times between birth and adulthood; then the brain loses weight by about 1 gram each year.

1 Brain and Body Weight

This scale shows brain weight as a percentage of body weight for selected backboned animals. At one extreme, Apatosaurus's brain was a mere one hundred-thousandth the weight of its enormous body. At the other end of the scale comes the spider monkey, with a better brain/body ratio than that of man.

A Spider monkey 4.8%.
B Sparrow 4.2%.
C Man 2.5%.
D Marmoset 1.4%.
E Dog 0.85%.
F Rat 0.48%.
G Elephant 0.2%.
H Whale 0.003%.
I Apatosaurus 0.001%.

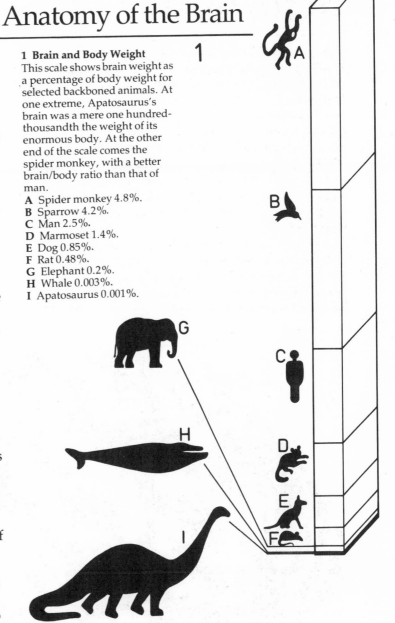

2 Human Brain Weights

This diagram shows the brain weights of three famous writers whose brains were weighed on death and compares them with extreme and average brain weights for humans.

a Heaviest known human brain 2049g.
b Jonathan Swift 2000g.
c Ivan Turgenev 2000g.
d Average man 1349g.
e Average women 1206g.
f Anatole France 1017g.
g Some microcephalics 300g.

2

● = 250g (8.8oz)

©DIAGRAM

The Parts of the Brain

The brain grows from the top end of the spinal cord as a crown of leaves sprouts from a cabbage stalk. To use another plant analogy, the parts making up the brain form layers somewhat like the layers of an onion. These two pages name and show the main parts of the brain and some of its associated structures. The brain has three parts: the forebrain (formed mostly by the cerebral hemispheres); the midbrain (the top of the brainstem); and the hindbrain, formed by the cerebellum and the remaining parts of the brainstem. The cerebrum consists of two huge hemispheres united by the corpus callosum, a fibrous band of tissue which also carries nerve tracts from one hemisphere to the other. The cerebrum sprawls up, out and over from the midbrain, masking the other regions of the brain. Its functions justify its relatively colossal size, for the cerebrum is the seat of our intelligence and memory – the place where we perceive, remember, think and take decisions.

Deep inside the cerebrum lie other forebrain structures doing similarly vital jobs. One of the most important units is the thalamus, located in the middle of the brain above the brainstem. The thalamus hands on information from the senses to the cerebrum and sends instructions from the cerebrum out to the body's muscles.

Below the thalamus lies a small, astonishingly versatile nerve cluster called the hypothalamus. This acts as an essential coordinator of the central nervous system; plays a crucial part in our emotions; and controls basic life processes, most of which we never even notice.

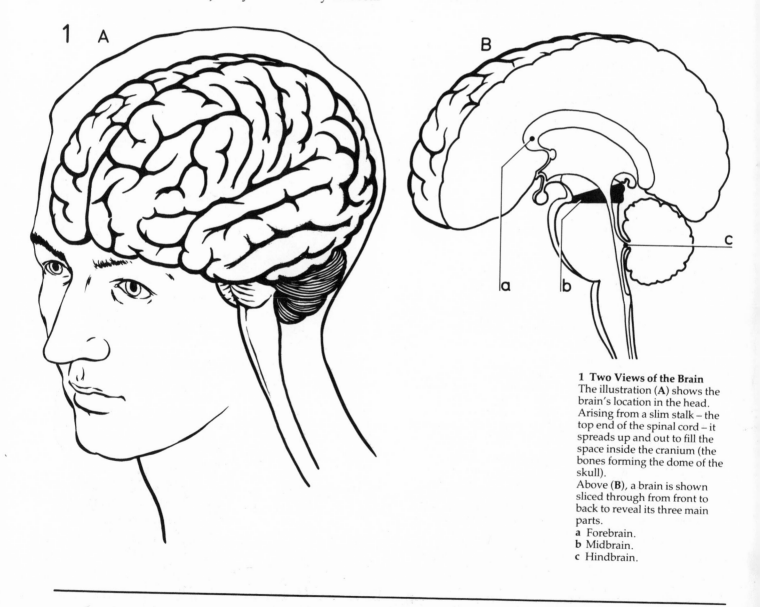

1 Two Views of the Brain
The illustration (**A**) shows the brain's location in the head. Arising from a slim stalk – the top end of the spinal cord – it spreads up and out to fill the space inside the cranium (the bones forming the dome of the skull).
Above (**B**), a brain is shown sliced through from front to back to reveal its three main parts.
a Forebrain.
b Midbrain.
c Hindbrain.

Two multiple structures complete this brief preview of the forebrain. Crowning the thalamus are the basal ganglia, four neuron clusters that help to regulate the body's movements.

This structure overlaps the limbic system, for both share a nerve knot known as the amygdala. The limbic system largely controls emotions and behavior, although part of it seems crucial for learning and short-term memory.

The midbrain, which lies below the forebrain, is the relatively narrow and short top of a bulging stalk of nerve fibers and nuclei called the brainstem. Much of the midbrain's work involves serving as a relay station for sensory impulses.

Below the midbrain comes the hindbrain. This includes the broad pons, and narrower medulla – the two lowest sections of the brainstem. Both have links with special sensors and carry vital pathways to and from the spinal cord.

The pons also provides a foothold for the cerebellum. Largest region of the hindbrain, and second largest structure in the brain, this bulges out and down behind the pons, back into the skull where part of the cerebrum overhangs it. The cerebellum is the great coordinator of complex movements of the body, especially the limbs.

Besides the structures briefly described above, the brain contains important subdivisions that we shall deal with later.

Within the brain lie fluid-filled cavities called ventricles, and on the brain's surface are meninges and blood vessels – structures providing essential support and nourishment.

2

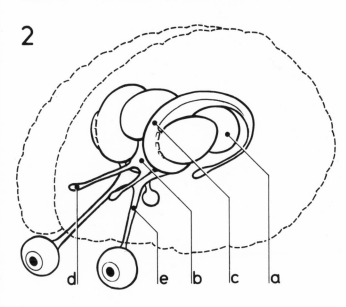

3

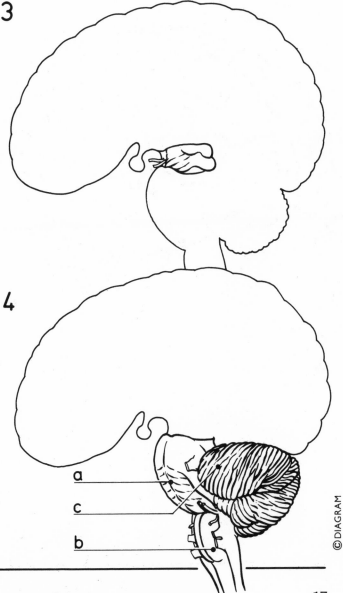

4

2 Forebrain Regions
Most of the forebrain is made up of two cerebral hemispheres, shown here in outline only. Inside lie other forebrain structures, most paired. They include:
a Thalamus.
b Hypothalamus.
c Basal ganglia.
d Olfactory lobes (part of the limbic system, not shown).
e Optic nerves.

3 Midbrain
Technically one of the three main regions of the brain, the midbrain forms no more than the shortest, highest section of the brainstem.

4 Hindbrain
The hindbrain embraces all brain structures below the midbrain. These are the pons and medulla in the brainstem proper and the cerebellum, which sprouts backward, behind the pons.
a Pons.
b Medulla oblongata.
c Cerebellum.

©DIAGRAM

The Cerebrum

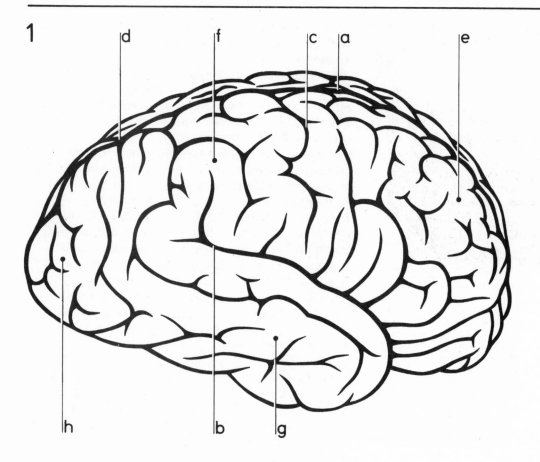

1

d   f   c   a   e

h   b   g

1 Cerebral Hemispheres
Here we show the right cerebral hemisphere viewed from the side. Labels indicate the main fissures, or sulci, and the lobes into which these help to divide each cerebral hemisphere.
a Longitudinal fissure between both hemispheres.
b Lateral fissure (fissure of Sylvius).
c Central fissure (fissure of Rolando).
d Parietal-Occipital fissure.
e Frontal lobe.
f Parietal lobe.
g Temporal lobe.
h Occipital lobe.

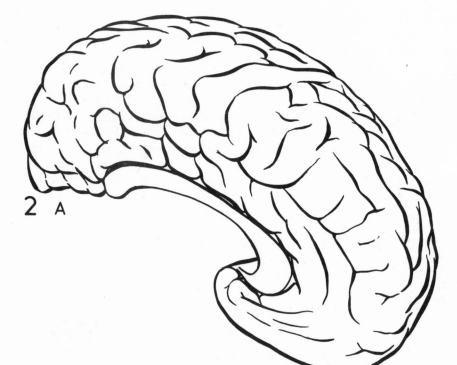

2 A

2 How a Hemisphere Grows
A This illustration shows a cerebral hemisphere viewed from its inner side, with part of the corpus callosum that joins the hemisphere to its neighbor.
B This diagram shows how the hemisphere (left) gained its curved shape. It grew forward, up, around, down, forward again, and then doubled back on itself to produce the lateral fissure between old and new regions of growth.

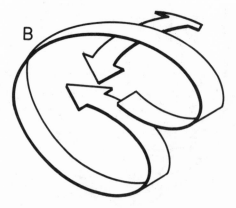

B

MOUNT MARY COLLEGE LIBRARY
Milwaukee, Wisconsin 53222

Anatomy of the Brain

3

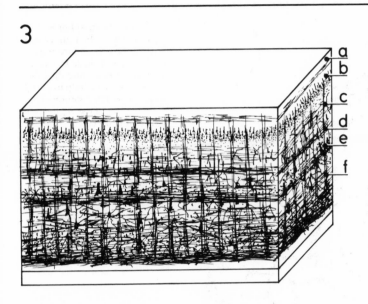

3 The Layered Cortex
The thin "bark" forming the cerebral cortex comprises six layers, shown (above) much enlarged. Some layers consist of distinctively shaped cells.
a (Outer) molecular layer.
b External granular layer.
c Outer pyramidal layer.
d Internal granular layer.
e Ganglionic layer.
f Multiform layer.

4 Cerebrum in Cross-Section
A section across the middle of both cerebral hemispheres shows their main internal features.
a Lateral fissure.
b Cerebral cortex.
c White matter.
d Longitudinal fissure.
e Ventricle (internal cavity).
f Inner forebrain centers.

4

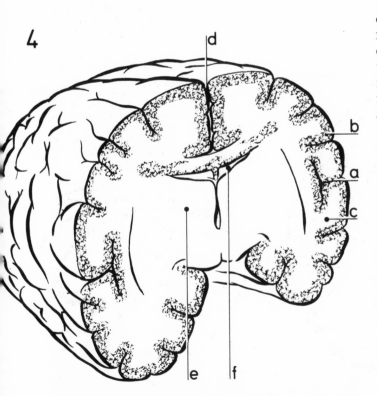

The giant wrinkled "walnut" of the cerebrum makes up seven-tenths of the entire nervous system.

At first glance, its wrinkles seem pointless and haphazard. In fact they enormously enlarge the surface area of brain that can be crammed inside the skull, and it is the surface layer that largely gives the brain intelligence.

Then, too, not every sulcus (fissure) or gyrus (ridge) is there by chance. Some figure in all our brains because of how these develop. The two lateral fissures and parieto-occipital fissures (one on each side) are constant features. Lateral fissures got there as the forebrain grew out, up, around, down, then back, in semihelix fashion, leaving crevices where new growth overlaps old. Each brain is split lengthwise down the middle by a deep rift – the longitudinal fissure. This valley divides the cerebrum into two almost identical cerebral hemispheres, united only deep down, near the center of the brain.

Identifying major fissures has helped anatomists divide each cerebral hemisphere into the frontal, occipital, temporal and parietal lobes – each named for the main skull bone that covers it. These landmarks help us to map the surface of the brain; but the lobes by no means exactly match brain areas designed for different tasks.

The cerebral surface misleads in other ways. A slice cut through one hemisphere shows that the gray matter making up the surface forms only a thin cortex ("bark") nowhere deeper than 4.5mm (less than one quarter of an inch). Amazingly, this fragile sheath contains perhaps 8000 million nerve cells, of several types, arranged in six layers, and interlinked by 10,000 miles (16,000km) of fibers for each cubic inch (16cm³). The cortex needs its rich cellular endowment, for the higher centers of the brain lodge here.

Below the gray matter of the cortex lies a far thicker white matter layer, colored by the fatty sheaths that clothe its nerve-cell fibers.

White matter includes hundreds of millions of nerve fibers uniting different regions of the cerebrum. There are three types of connection. Association fibers link different parts of the same hemisphere. Projection fibers fan out from the brainstem to all parts of the cerebrum. A dense mass of commissural ("joining") fibers builds the corpus callosum ("hard body") – the bridge 4 inches (10cm) long that joins both hemispheres.

© DIAGRAM

83-1716

The Basal Ganglia and Limbic System

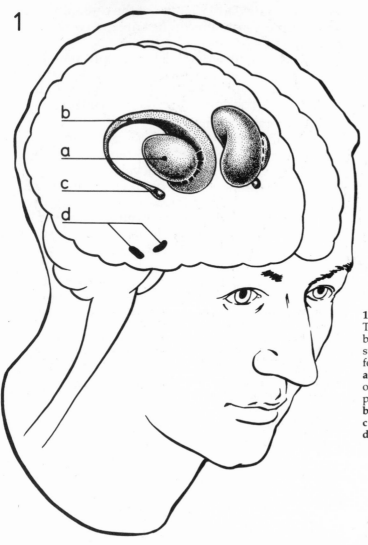

1 The Basal Ganglia
The paired structures of the basal ganglia form one of the special systems deep within the forebrain.
a Lentiform nucleus (made up of the globus pallidus and the putamen).
b Caudate nucleus.
c Amygdala.
d Substantia nigra.

Some brain structures form groups that work as special systems. Two such groups are the basal ganglia and the limbic system. After the thalamus and hypothalamus, these are the innermost layers of that "animal onion" the forebrain.

The four nerve-cell clusters of the basal ganglia or "nerve knots" help to handle physical movements by relaying information from the cerebral cortex to the brainstem and cerebellum. The system's core is the lentiform ("lens-shaped") nucleus, made of the globus pallidus ("pale ball") and intriguingly-named putamen ("that which drops when a tree is pruned"). The caudate ("tail-shaped") nucleus wraps around the first two as a tail, ending in the amygdala ("almond"). Nearby, a cerebral cortex strip earned the name claustrum ("barrier") for its supposed resemblance to a wall outside the lentiform nucleus. Sometimes included with the

basal ganglia are two other structures – one near the thalamus, the other in the brainstem. Their streaked appearance, when seen sliced through, explains their collective name of corpus striatum ("striped body").

Encircling the brainstem with a "wishbone" structure, the limbic system is a mini brain handling emotions and involved in memory. This system's close links with the olfactory tracts at first fooled scientists into calling the whole complex the rhinencephalon ("nose brain"), until they realized that some animals with limbic systems could scarcely smell at all.

Limbic ("bordering") is a better name, as this system's cortex, tucked in around the brainstem, bounds the neck between the diencephalon ("between brain") – the old, innermost part of the forebrain – and the telencephalon ("end brain") –

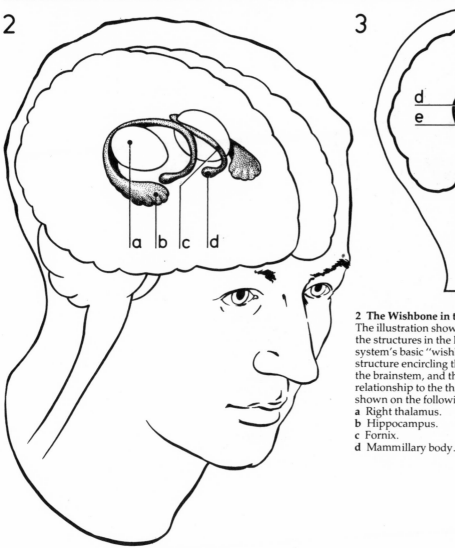

2

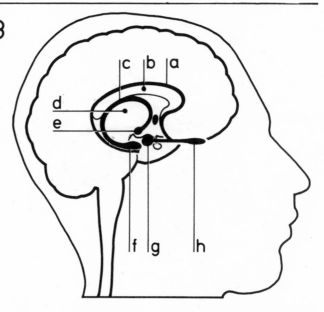

3

2 The Wishbone in the Brain
The illustration shows some of the structures in the limbic system's basic "wishbone" structure encircling the top of the brainstem, and their relationship to the thalami shown on the following page.
a Right thalamus.
b Hippocampus.
c Fornix.
d Mammillary body.

3 The Limbic System
The limbic system is made up of a complex of curved structures which, in side view, appear to nest one inside the other.
a Supracallosal gyrus.
b Corpus callosum.
c Fornix.
d Thalamus.
e Mammillary body.
f Hippocampus.
g Amygdala.
h Olfactory bulb.

the newest forebrain region, comprising most of the cerebral hemispheres.

Called archicortex ("original bark") and paleocortex ("old bark"), regions of the limbic system's outer "skin" are older in evolutionary terms than the neocortex ("new bark") covering most of the forebrain. Indeed man's limbic system shows little difference from that of primitive mammals – hence its nickname: "old mammalian brain."

Fanciful names identify items belonging to or linked with the system's basic wishbone structure. Each prong features an S-shaped hippocampus ("sea horse"), above a gyrus and flanked at one end by an amygdala. Both prongs of the wishbone are tied together by bundles of nerve fibers belonging to the fornix ("arch") and anterior commissure ("forward joining"). The septum pellucidum

("transparent wall") juts up between both prongs near the wishbone's far end. Here, at the prong tips, bulge mammillary ("breastlike") bodies. Sweeping around the whole wishbone are the curves of the two cingulate gyri ("girdling convolutions") – a pair of cerebral ridges, one in each hemisphere.

Impulses speed through the limbic system's own internal pathways, through paths to other forebrain regions, and to the cerebellum. Triggered or modulated by these signals, limbic structures arouse or temper feelings that range from joy to misery and love to hate, as well as helping to control memory. Later, we shall examine in more detail how aspects of the system operate.

©DIAGRAM

The 'Between-Brain' Centers

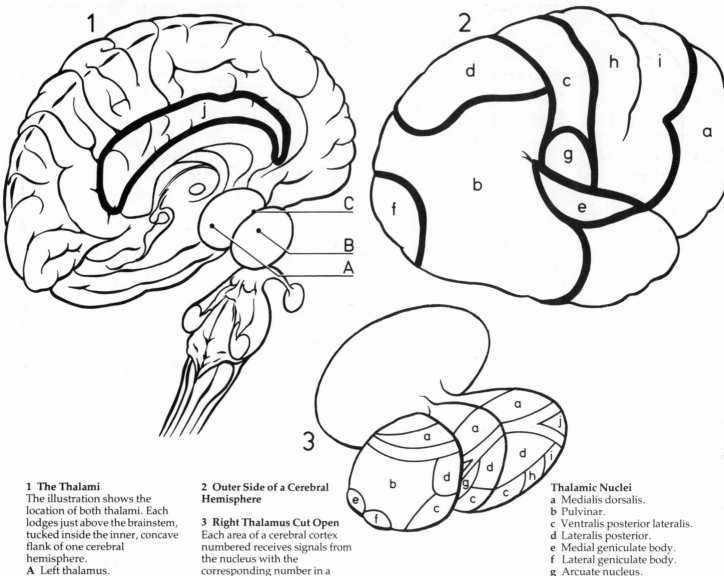

1 The Thalami
The illustration shows the location of both thalami. Each lodges just above the brainstem, tucked inside the inner, concave flank of one cerebral hemisphere.
A Left thalamus.
B Right thalamus.
C Interthalamic connection.

2 Outer Side of a Cerebral Hemisphere

3 Right Thalamus Cut Open
Each area of a cerebral cortex numbered receives signals from the nucleus with the corresponding number in a thalamus.

Thalamic Nuclei
a Medialis dorsalis.
b Pulvinar.
c Ventralis posterior lateralis.
d Lateralis posterior.
e Medial geniculate body.
f Lateral geniculate body.
g Arcuate nucleus.
h Lateralis dorsalis.
i Ventralis anterior.
j Anterior nuclear group.

Thalamus, hypothalamus, pituitary gland and pineal gland are features in the diencephalon or "between brain," the region deep in the forebrain between brainstem and cerebral hemispheres. The two thalami ("deep chambers") are egg-shaped masses of gray matter astride the top of the brainstem and joined across the brain's midline by the massa intermedia ("intermediate mass"), a tract of fibers. The thalami are major integrators of information flowing in from sensory organs to the the cerebral cortex. All sensory signals pass this way. In each thalamus lie nuclei handling special types of signal. For instance, the ventrobasal complex takes information fed in from the body via the spinal cord; the lateral geniculate ("bent") body receives optic-tract input from the eyes; the medial geniculate body takes signals from the ears. After analysis, each type of signal speeds on to a specific part of the cerebral cortex. But input from the brainstem's reticular formation is beamed out to all parts of the cortex.

Between thalamus and brainstem lies the tiny hypothalamus ("under the thalamus"). No larger than a thumb tip and weighing only one quarter of an ounce (14g), the hypothalamus performs more kinds of task than any other brain structure of its size. It has four main areas of nuclei: preoptic, anterior ("forward"), middle and posterior.

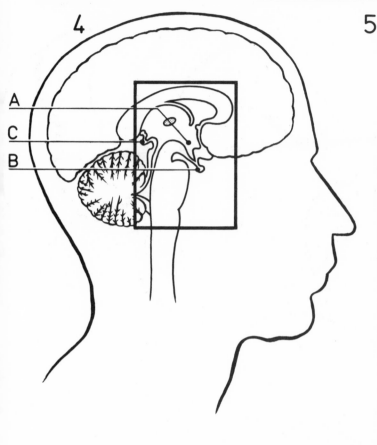

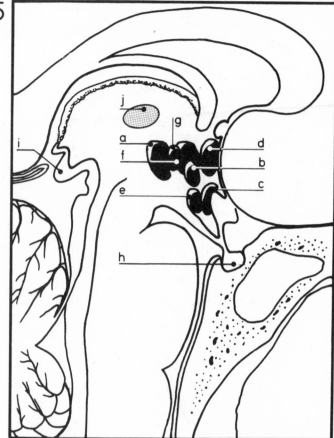

4 Three Centers
This diagram shows the locations of hypothalamus, pituitary gland and pineal gland between the brainstem and cerebral hemispheres.
A Hypothalamus.
B Pituitary gland.
C Pineal gland.

5 Hypothalamic Regions
This enlarged view depicts seven hypothalamic regions, each with a specific function.
a Posterior: sex drive
b Anterior: water balance.
c Supraoptic: water balance.
d Preoptic: heat control.
e Ventromedial: hunger.
f Dorsomedial: aggression.
g Dorsal: pleasure.

Pituitary Gland
The pituitary gland (**h**) is almost an appendage of the hypothalamus, which in fact controls the pituitary's storage and output of hormones.

Pineal Gland
The cone-shaped pineal gland (**i**) is connected by nerve pathways to the eyes, and it shows surprising sensitivity to light. Its position in relation to the thalami can be seen from the site of the interthalamic connection (**j**).

Between them, these special regions regulate body temperature, control thirst and appetite, and influence blood pressure, sexual behavior, aggression, fear and sleep.
Like any forebrain structure, the hypothalamus liaises closely with other areas, especially the limbic system, and controls the pituitary gland. The pituitary ("slime") gland owes its misleading name to an old notion that nasal secretions originated in this pea-sized nerve center hung in a bony dip at the base of the skull. More aptly called "leader of the endocrine orchestra," the pituitary yields hormones that influence other glands, regulating vital bodily activities. This gland is really two glands in one. The anterior pituitary yields hormones affecting (among other things) growth, sexual development, and food conversion into energy. Its overactivity produces giants; underactivity, dwarfs. The posterior pituitary stores hypothalamus-produced hormones regulating urine output, and so helps conserve water in the body; it also influences oxytocin production, and the process of lactation.
Projecting down above the back of the brainstem, the pinecone-shaped pineal gland poses an enigma. People once considered it a vestigial third eye. Now, research suggests rather a light-sensitive clock affecting sleep and sex glands.

©DIAGRAM

The Brainstem

The brainstem jutting up from the spinal cord is less than 3 inches (7.6cm) long. The brain's root and core, it serves as highway for motor and sensory nerve fibers, initiator of action in higher centers of the brain, controller of consciousness, and regulator of essential life processes.
Found in all reptiles and their bird and mammal descendants, the vital if primitive brainstem is sometimes called the reptilian brain. This structure's three main sections are medulla, pons and midbrain. Above the spinal cord, you come first to the medulla oblongata ("rather long marrow"), a fibrous section of stem, 1 inch (2.5cm) long, resembling no more than a thick extension of the spinal cord. Part telephone exchange, this links the higher brain centers with senses served by the eighth, ninth, tenth, eleventh, and twelfth cranial nerves – all springing from knots of nerve cells inside the medulla. Other groups of nerve cells keep heart and lungs working.

Where medulla meets spinal cord, 900,000 of the million nerve fibers in each of the so-called corticospinal tracts switch sides in a grand crossing over – the corticospinal decussation. Bundles of sensory nerves from the left side of the body have shifted to the right side of the brain, while bundles of motor nerves from the right side of the brain shift to the left side of the body, and vice versa. Thus each side of the brain controls the opposite side of the body.
The pons or "bridge" is a bulge of white matter 1 inch (2.5cm) broad bridging the space between midbrain and medulla. Interwoven with longitudinal nerve fibers, thick bundles of

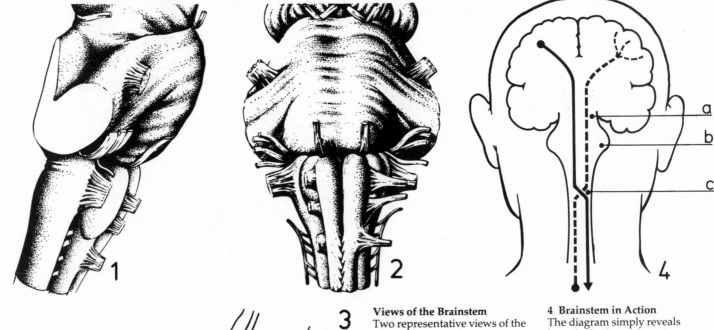

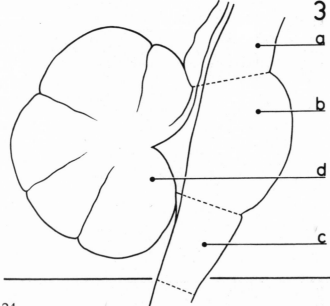

Views of the Brainstem
Two representative views of the brainstem show also nerve fibers that end or start at this relay station and control center for vital life processes.
1 Representative side view.
2 Representative front view.
3 Diagram of side view to show the brainstem's three main parts:
a Midbrain.
b Pons.
c Medulla oblongata.
d The cerebellum, behind the pons, is not strictly a part of the brainstem, and we describe it separately on the following pages.

4 Brainstem in Action
The diagram simply reveals how the brainstem serves as a relay for signals that pass between cerebral hemispheres above and spinal cord below. Broken lines show sensory signals flowing in to the brain. Solid lines show motor impulses flowing out from brain to muscles. Note the crossing in the medulla, so that each side of the brain deals with the opposite side of the body.
a Midbrain.
b Pons.
c Medulla oblongata.

transverse fibers sprout from the pons to the cerebellum. Also, four of the twelve cranial nerves have their nuclei (relay stations) here, including the large trigeminal nerve.

Less than 1 inch (2.5cm) long, the midbrain at the top of the brainstem is far smaller than the forebrain or the hindbrain. Sensory impulses track through this relay station, and here two cranial nerves have their roots. The midbrain governs some reflex muscle activity; for instance, adjusting the size and movements of the pupil of the eye. Deep in the brainstem, from medulla to midbrain, runs the reticular formation. This thimble-sized thicket of small nerve cells and short fibers rules consciousness. Even when we sleep, this hidden watchdog stays on guard, ready to alert the forebrain if the senses signal "danger."

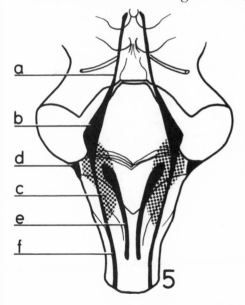

5 Sensory Nuclei
These brainstem nerve centers receive sensations from specific sensory nerves. Nuclei a, b and f between them receive signals from the face, mouth and sinuses.
a Nucleus of the mesencephalic tract (cranial nerve V).
b Sensory nucleus of the trigeminal nerve (V).
c Vestibular nucleus, dealing with balance (VIII).
d Cochlear nucleus, dealing with sound (VIII).
e Viscerosensory nucleus, keyed to tongue and internal organs (IX, X).
f Nucleus of spinal tract (V).

6 Motor Nuclei
These brainstem nerve centers transmit orders to muscles.
a Edinger-Westphal nucleus supplying parts of the eye.
b Oculomotor nerve nucleus.
c Nucleus of the trochlear nerve, working an eye muscle.
d Motor nucleus of the trigeminal nerve, working the muscles that chew.
e Nucleus of the abducens, controlling an eye muscle.
f Nucleus of the facial nerve, working facial muscles.
g Upper salivatory nucleus.
h Lower salivatory nucleus.
i Nucleus ambiguus, motor nucleus of the vagus nerve, supplying internal organs.
j Dorsal nucleus of the vagus nerve.
k Nucleus of hypoglossal nerve, for tongue muscles.
l Nucleus of the accessory nerve, for shoulder muscles.

7 Side View
This schematic side view of the brainstem shows the same sensory and motor nuclei as in the diagram to the left, with tallying annotation. Among structures not shown is the important reticular formation, which runs up through the brainstem.

©DIAGRAM

The Cerebellum

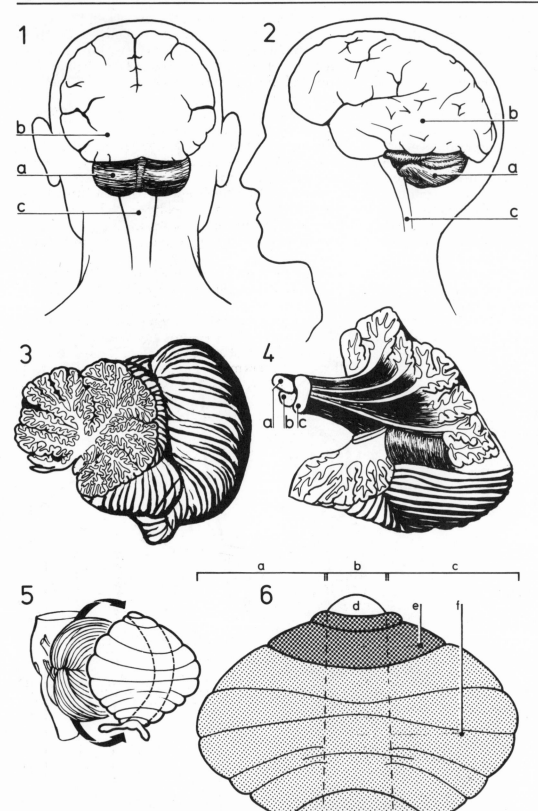

The Cerebellum

The cerebellum serves valuable roles in maintaining posture and adjusting muscle movements. Much of its work involves checking jerky movement, and it may act as a kind of automatic pilot when we perform learned functions like driving or brushing our teeth. Two views of the head show the cerebellum's position at the back of the brain.

1 Rear view:
a Cerebellum.
b Cerebrum.
c Brainstem.
2 Side view:
a Cerebellum.
b Cerebrum.
c Brainstem.

Cerebellar Sections

Two cut-away views reveal the cerebellum's internal arbor vitae ("tree of life") form.
3 A side view with the cerebellum shown cut through the middle.
4 Part of one of the two hemispheres flanking the cerebellum's central vermis. Letters show sections arising from the three fibrous pillars (peduncles) that attach the cerebellum to the brainstem.
a Superior peduncle.
b Inferior peduncle.
c Middle peduncle.

The Cerebellum Mapped

5 The convoluted mass of the cerebellum is shown in its normal position at the back of the brainstem. Arrows show how the organ is schematically 'unfolded' to identify its structures.
6 Unfolded, the cerebellum areas can be mapped:
a Left hemisphere.
b Vermis.
c Right hemisphere.
d Evolutionarily old lobes, concerned with balance.
e "Old" lobes receiving data about muscle sensations.
f Evolutionarily young lobes receiving information from the cerebral cortex concerning central control.

About 11 per cent of the entire weight of the brain is in the structure called the cerebellum ("little brain"). Its main work is vetting data fed in from the muscles, joints, tendons and inner ear and acting on this information to adjust posture and coordinate muscular movements ordered by the cerebrum. The cerebellum may also influence emotional development.

Just how much coordination matters to us can be judged from the cerebellum's size, which has more than trebled in the last million years. In the whole brain, only the cerebrum is larger.

The huge size of man's cerebellum contrasts sharply with that of primitive backboned animals like amphibians, in which the cerebellum is relatively small and underdeveloped.

Bulging from the back of the brainstem into the back of the skull, the cerebellum looks rather like a small version of the cerebrum. Its gray surface is so deeply wrinkled that all but 15 per cent of it is hidden in the leaflike folds. But the cerebellum's structure is laid down more precisely than the cerebrum's.

Seen from below, the "little brain" has three main parts: a central, somewhat grublike vermis ("worm"), flanked by two winglike lateral hemispheres. The whole structure is doubled over, like an accordian, with both ends turned in as if to meet. Unfolded, a cerebellar cortex would measure 47 inches (120cm) by 6½ inches (17cm). Seen that way, the cerebellum consists of parallel pleats or lobes. The largest lobes lie in the middle. These mainly handle orders sent out from the cerebral cortex. The smallest pleats – in evolutionary terms the oldest parts – link up with the spinal cord and inner ear.

Three pairs of fibrous pillars, the peduncles ("little feet"), link the cerebellum to the brainstem. The inferior (lower), middle, and superior (upper) peduncles respectively spring from the medulla, pons, and midbrain, and between them carry all the traffic of nerve impulses that commutes between the cerebellum, cerebral cortex and spinal cord.

Cutting through a cerebellum shows the fanning out and funneling in of white nerve fibers taking signals to and from the gray matter of the cerebellum's outer surface. Fibers bringing signals in outnumber fibers sending signals out by three to one. But the most amazing feature is the middle of three cell layers making up the gray matter. Each of this layer's so-called Purkinje cells can contact no fewer than 100,000 other fibers, making more connections than any other type of brain cell can achieve.

Cells of the Cerebellum
Careful mapping has revealed numerous cerebellar cell types. Here, a magnified section through a cerebellar convolution shows three layers, with the main cell types and their connections.
A Molecular layer.
B Purkinje cell layer.
C Granular layer.
a Parallel fibers.
b Stellate cell.
c Basket cell.
d Axons.
e Purkinje cell.
f Climbing fiber.
g Golgi cell.
h Granule.
i Mossy fiber.

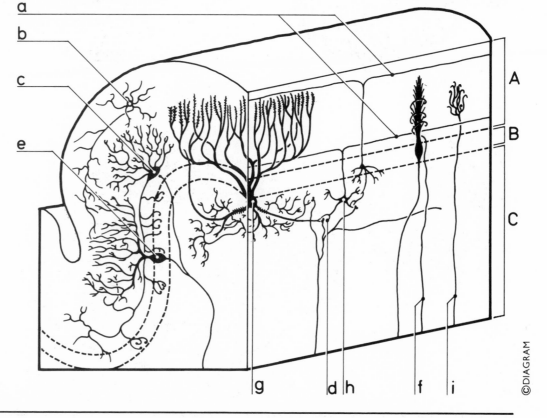

©DIAGRAM

Protection and Nourishment

Man's brain is a fragile, ravenous organ. Five hard and soft layers and two fluids provide a lifetime's protection and nourishment. From the outside inward the brain is shielded by layers of skin, bone and three membranes called meninges.

The body's thickest skin is the scalp, which includes layers of fat and connective tissue. Hair normally sprouts thickly from the scalp and helps to insulate the top of the head.

Below the scalp lies the skull, formed of 22 bones, in adults fused together along rigid zigzag joints known as sutures. Eight of these bones make up the strong, dome-shaped cranium housing the brain. The two bony layers of the skull guard the delicate brain from all but the harshest blows. By enclosing its soft, rubbery form, the skull also helps to give the brain its shape.

Beneath the skull lie the three meninges that totally enclose the brain. The outer membrane is the tough, thick, leathery dura mater ("hard mother"). Directly below lies the arachnoid (Greek for "spider's web"). A web of tissues from this thin membrane crosses a gap filled with cerebrospinal fluid and connects the arachnoid with the third and innermost membrane. This so-called pia mater ("soft mother") hugs the brain's outer surface and supplies it with blood.

Each minute over 1½ US pints (about 800ml) of blood flows through the brain. Accounting for only one-fiftieth of the body's weight, the brain receives one-fifth of its total supply of blood and oxygen. Awake or asleep, the brain uses oxygen to "burn" up glucose – a food also supplied by the blood. Each day the brain takes about 400 kilocalories,

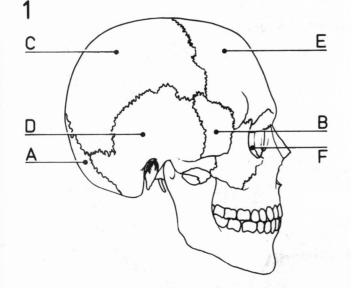

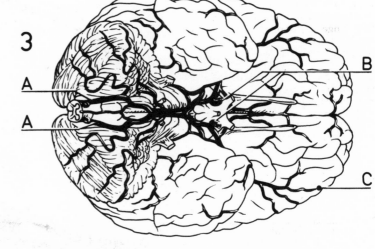

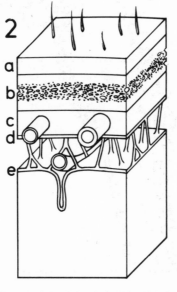

1 The Cranium
The brain is shielded by eight fused skull bones (above) that combine to form the cranium.

A Occipital bone, a bowl-shaped ("against head") bone at the back of the head.

B Sphenoid bone, a "wedge-shaped" bone at the base of the skull.

C Parietal bones, two "wall" bones at the top and sides of the head.

D Temporal bones, two bones "of the temples," ie above the ears.

E Frontal bone, the bone forming the forehead.

F Ethmoid bone, a bone "like a sieve." This lies behind the nose and is pierced to take olfactory nerve bundles.

2 Five-Ply Protection
The cross section (left) shows the five layers that guard the brain and help to shape it.

a Scalp, with hair, skin, fat and other tissue.

b Cranium, the part of the skull housing the brain. Its inner network of bony struts and dome-like shape give this structure its strength.

c Dura mater, the tough, unstretchable outer membrane embracing the brain.

d Arachnoid, an elastic "skin" enclosing the so-called subarachnoid space.

e Pia mater, a thin "skin" that clings closely to the brain's irregular surface.

3 Blood Supply
The diagram (above) shows part of the brain's blood supply. This comes from two vertebral arteries (**A**) that reach the brain through a large hole in the base of the skull, and two internal carotid arteries (**B**) that reach the brain via other holes low down in the skull. Many arteries branch out and follow valleys in the brain's wrinkled surface (**C**). Most used blood drains out of the brain via the internal jugular veins at the base of the skull.

equal to one-fifth of all food required by a sedentary woman.

Our brains need to be greedy. Unable to store oxygen or glucose, they depend for survival on an uninterrupted blood supply. Ten seconds' break in the flow brings unconsciousness. A few minutes' oxygen starvation can kill, or transform a genius into a mindless zombie. Yet the brain's requirement for nourishment can vary, within limits. A slackened flow marks increased physical effort, while two hours' intense mental effort calls for no more extra glucose than you can get by eating just one peanut.

Besides nourishing the brain, blood provides it with a watery cushion of cerebrospinal fluid (CSF), produced from the blood chiefly by choroid plexuses – clusters of tiny "fingers" lining parts of

the ventricles, four linked cavities deep inside the brain. The fluid fills these cavities, and flows via special ducts around the brain's outer rim before being reabsorbed into the blood. Thus the brain floats in a bath that may effectively reduce its weight by 20 times. This surrounding fluid buffers the brain against shock and makes turning or nodding the head an effortless act instead of excruciating torment. Cerebrospinal fluid also protects the spinal cord. In fact only one-fifth of an average adult's normal quota of CSF lies in the brain. Cerebrospinal fluid pressure varies harmlessly with body posture. Rarely, a dangerous build-up may occur, requiring medical aid.

4 Cerebrospinal Fluid
CSF appears and flows around the brain as shown here.
A Choroid plexus, masses of tiny "fingers" that produce cerebrospinal fluid.
B Lateral ventricle. (The brain has two such cavities.)
C Third ventricle.
D Fourth ventricle.
E Subarachnoid space through which cerebrospinal fluid circulates around the brain.
F Arachnoid granulations (one shown below enlarged) These act as valves that let cerebrospinal fluid escape to venous sinuses.
G Venous sinus. Such channels between layers of the dura mater carry off used blood and cerebrospinal fluid.

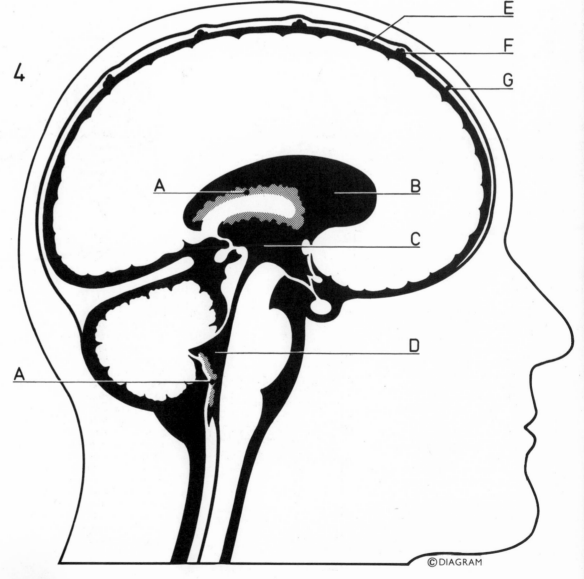

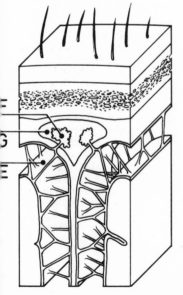

©DIAGRAM

Chapter 2

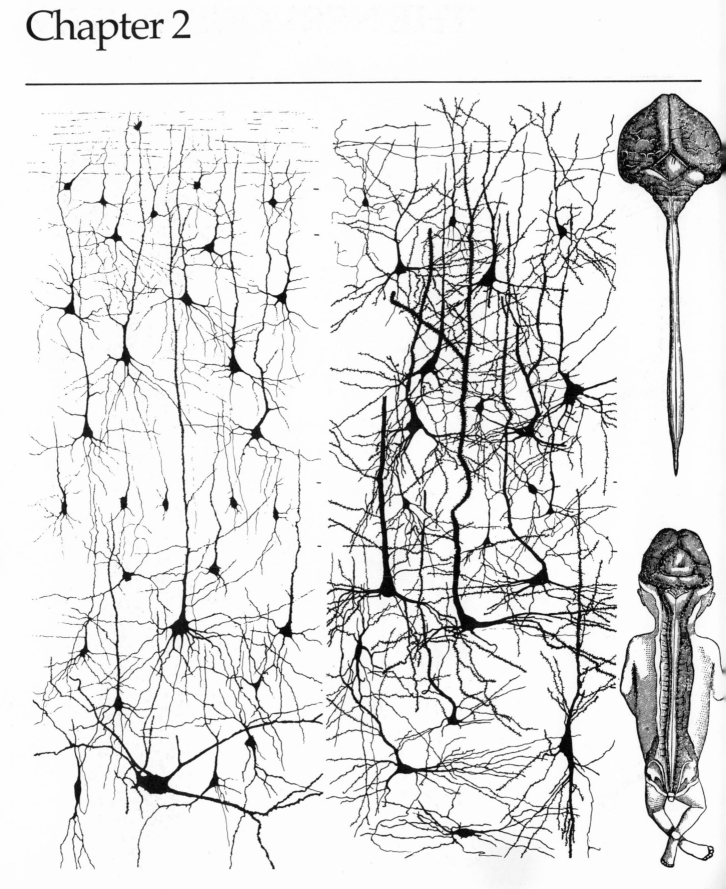

THE NERVOUS SYSTEM

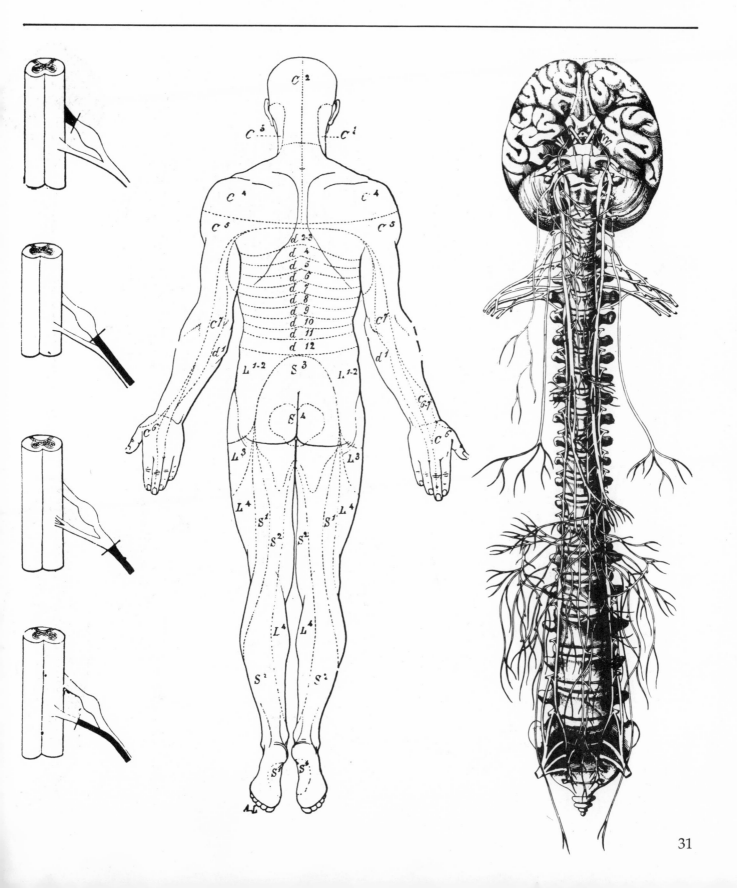

The Central Nervous System

Disconnected from input and output, a computer's control unit would be useless. Similarly, your brain depends on nerves that wire it up to the body's sense organs and muscles. This chapter looks beyond the brain to the broader wiring of the nervous system, then investigates nerve cells and how these send their signals to and fro.

In evolutionary terms, the brain itself is just a complex outgrowth of the spinal cord. Indeed, both make up the body's central nervous system – its key roles being receiving sensory data, making decisions, and sending out commands to muscles. Compared with the convoluted brain, the spinal cord appears a simple structure, in keeping with its relatively lowly functions: performing reflex actions and transmitting nervous impulses to and from the brain. But cord and brain share some important features, and though the cord may be more primitive, physiologists have by no means yet unraveled all its operations.

A soft, curved cylinder, the spinal cord descends inside the backbone for about 18 inches (46cm) from a big hole at the base of the skull, where the cord's upper end joins the brainstem, to the level of the first lumbar ("apron for the loins") vertebra, well above the bottom of the spine. The cord bulges at those levels from which nerves branch off to supply the arms and legs. But below the first lumbar vertebra it continues downward as no more than a fine thread, tethered to the back of the coccyx (loosely meaning "cuckoo's bill"), the tail end of the backbone.

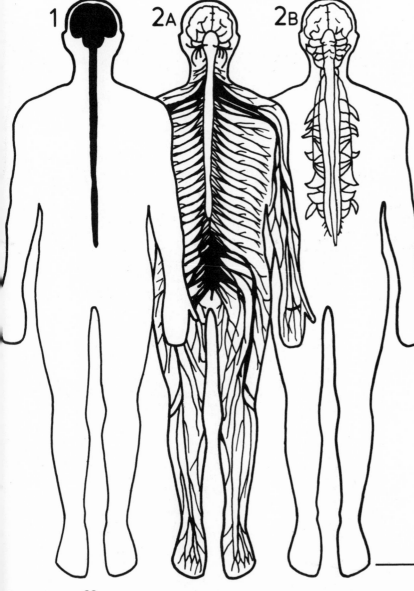

Two Nervous Systems
The body's nervous system consists of two main parts that act as a unit.
1 Central nervous system (CNS). The brain and spinal cord form the body's control center, receiving and transmitting information via the peripheral nervous system (PNS). The PNS is divided into two sections:
2A The somatic nervous system is concerned with conscious actions and reflexes and supplies parts of the body under voluntary control.
2B The autonomic nervous system controls unconscious activities such as heartbeat and breathing.

3 The Spine
A section through the spine (below) shows how the spinal cord (**a**) passes through the vertebrae (**b**). The cord is protected by the meninges (**c**). Nerves (**d**) belonging to the PNS leave the cord at intervals.

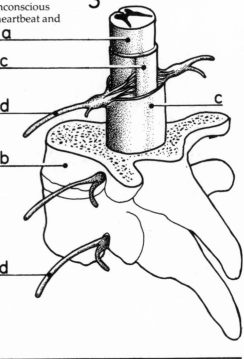

Arched bones of the vertebrae enclose and shield the vulnerable cord. Inside this bony cave the cord is safety-wrapped by three membranes – continuations of the meninges that surround the brain. Similarly, a cerebrospinal fluid cushion surrounds the cord, protecting it from jarring. The spinal cord has a white outer layer of insulated nerve fibers which carry signals – some up, some down the cord. Enclosed by this white layer lies a butterfly-shaped gray section of the nerve cells that forms a fluted column running up inside the outer cord.

The butterfly's lower "wings," facing chest or belly, hold nerve fibers controlling muscles. Upper "wings," which face the back, contain cells receiving sensory signals from outside the spinal cord. Different areas inside the spinal cord affect different regions of the body.

At intervals along the cord, each wingtip sprouts a nerve root – four per "butterfly." From each wing, both roots join to form a mixed (part-sensory, part-motor) spinal nerve that exists from the spine through one of the two gaps in the bone between each pair of vertebrae.

The 31 pairs of spinal nerves roughly tally in number with the gaps available. But because the spine grows longer than the spinal cord, the cord's lower nerve roots get out of step with their exit holes and must grow far downward through the spinal canal before they can escape. The resulting fan of nerve roots in the lower spine creates the cauda equina ("horse's tail").

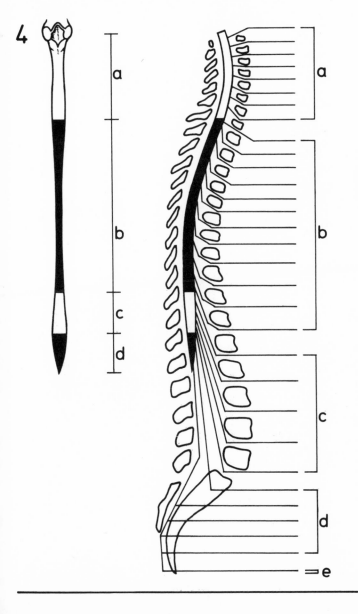

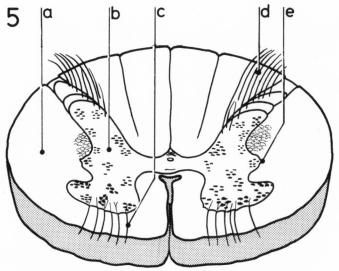

4 Spinal Nerves
The 31 pairs of nerves leaving the spinal cord (left) are divided into four main groups.
a 8 pairs of cervical nerves supply the throat, chest, arms and hands.
b 12 pairs of thoracic nerves supply the middle part of the body from the top of the breastbone to the bottom of the ribs and the abdomen.
c 5 pairs of lumbar nerves supply the front of the legs and the feet.
d 5 pairs of sacral nerves and the coccygeal nerve (**e**) supply the soles of the feet and the backs of the legs.

5 Spinal Cord
The spinal cord cross-section (above) shows the white matter (**a**) that conducts signals up and down the spinal cord and the butterfly-shaped gray matter (**b**) that transmits signals into and out of the cord. Nerves (**c**) arising from the part of the butterfly facing the front of the body carry outgoing signals that control muscles. Nerves (**d**) carrying sensory signals from the body's surface, and deeper structures such as muscles, enter the spinal cord at the back of the butterfly. The small projections (**e**) at either side contain nerve cells belonging to the autonomic nervous system.

© DIAGRAM

The Peripheral Nervous System

From brain and spinal cord, nerves divide and subdivide, supplying almost every cranny of the body. Anatomists have devised various methods of grouping these nerves that run outside the central nervous system. The simplest way of looking at them is to use the name "peripheral nerves" for all 12 pairs of cranial nerves projecting from the brain (though some are strictly speaking brain tracts) and all 31 pairs of nerves rooted in the spinal cord. The peripheral nerves in turn may be divided into two main groups making up the so-called somatic ("bodily") and autonomic ("self-regulating") nervous systems.

The somatic system features two kinds of nerves. Motor nerves branching from the central nervous system make muscles act on orders from the brain or spinal cord. Sensory nerves taking signals in the opposite direction home in on the central nervous system, bringing information from sensors in skin, eyes, tongue, nostrils, joints and muscles. Subconsciously bombarded by this artillery of information, we use the knowledge it brings about our posture and surroundings to control how we hold ourselves or move around.

The autonomic system serves the different function of automatically controlling glands and structures like the lungs, heart, blood vessels and pupils of the eyes. Linked with the spinal cord and brain's hypothalamus, this system is influenced by the central nervous system, but most people tend to think of it as beyond the brain's conscious control. In fact the autonomic system harks back

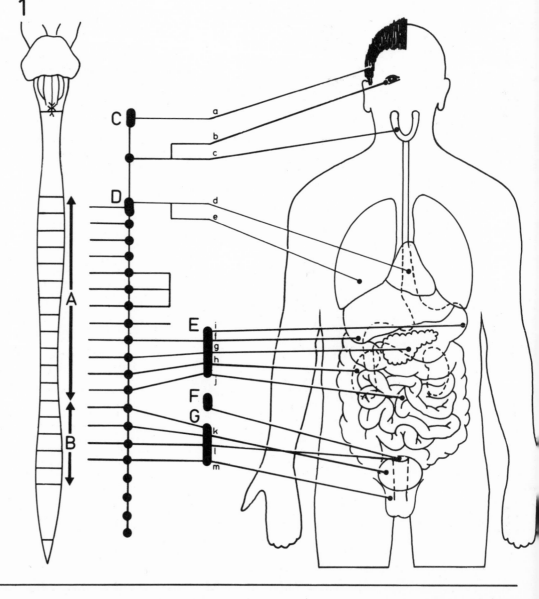

Autonomic Nervous System
The ANS regulates those activities over which we have no conscious control (involuntary activities). It is probably controlled by the hypothalamus and consists of two systems – the sympathetic and the parasympathetic, which work more or less in opposition.

1 Sympathetic System
Nerves work as a unit, dealing particularly with the body's reactions to emergency. In times of physical danger or stress, they cause sweating, increase blood pressure, and mobilize the body's systems for fight or flight. Nerves leave the thoracic (**A**) and lumbar (**B**) regions of the spinal cord and pass through a chain of nerve centers (ganglia) before reaching the part of the body they activate.

C Superior cervical ganglion is the nerve center supplying blood vessels of the head (**a**), the pupils of the eyes (**b**) and the salivary glands (**c**).

D Stellate ganglion supplies nerves that accelerate the action of the heart (**d**) and increase the respiratory power of the lungs (**e**).

E Celiac ganglion; nerves supply the liver (**f**), pancreas (**g**) and kidneys (**h**), and relax the muscular walls of the stomach (**i**) and intestines (**j**).

F Superior mesenteric ganglion.

G Inferior mesenteric ganglion supplies nerves to the bladder (**k**), rectum (**l**) and genitals (**m**).

hundreds of millions of years to our backboneless ancestors whose nervous system comprised two poorly integrated parts – one sensitive to stimuli outside the body, the other coping with events inside.

The autonomic nervous system consists of two sub-systems: the sympathetic and parasympathetic nervous systems. Each acts in opposition to the other. Springing from all but top and bottom of the spinal cord, nerve fibers of the sympathetic nervous system supply eyes, nose, salivary glands, heart, lungs, stomach, liver, kidneys, genitals and other glands or muscles. Output from the sympathetic nervous system steps up internal bodily activity, increasing heart rate, dilating pupils, and switching blood supply

from the intestines to the brain and muscles. The parasympathetic system serves most of the same organs as the sympathetic system. But nerves supplying organs as far down as the intestines are cranial nerves, sprouting from the brainstem. The rest – supplying bladder, kidneys and reproductive organs – spring from the bottom of the spinal cord. Unlike the sympathetic nervous system, the parasympathetic system puts a brake on heart rate, contracts pupils, and feeds blood away from brain and muscles to intestines. Normally the two opposing systems keep some kind of balance in the body. But, under stress, the sympathetic system dominates, while relaxation sees the parasympathetic system in command.

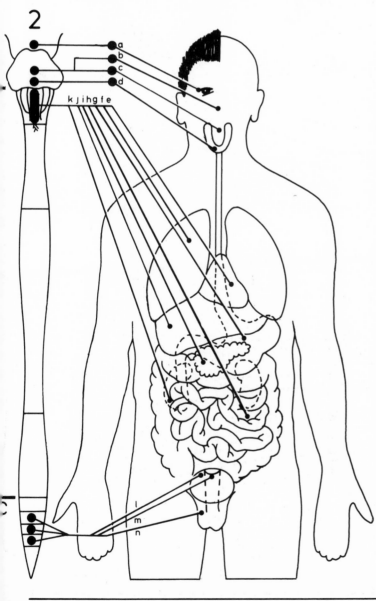

2

k j i h g f e

a
b
c
d

l
m
n

2 Parasympathetic System
Nerves work individually, stimulating muscles to work, producing digestive juices and generally keeping the body's systems ticking over at a steady, normal rate.
A Three cranial nerves contract the pupil of the eye (**a**), and supply the membranes of the nose (**b**) and palate (**c**), and the secretory parts of the salivary glands (**d**).
B A fourth cranial nerve splits up into many branches that slow the action of the heart (**e**) and lungs (**f**), increase the activity of the stomach (**g**) and intestines (**h**) and supply the pancreas (**i**), liver (**j**) and kidneys (**k**).
C Sacral nerves supply the bladder (**l**), rectum (**m**) and genitals (**n**).

3 Somatic Nerves
The diagram illustrates the paths of different types of message through the spinal cord. Somatic sensory fibers (**A**) bring messages from receptors in the skin, joints and striated muscle (**B**); somatic motor fibers (**C**) carry these to skeletal muscle (**D**). Visceral sensory fibers (**E**) carry messages from smooth muscle (**F**); visceral motor fibers (**G**) relay them back to smooth muscle and to glands (**H**).

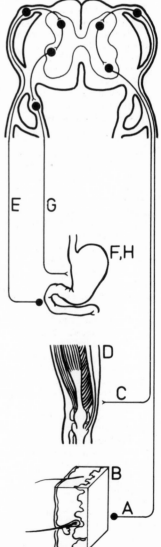

E   G

F,H

D

C

B

A

©DIAGRAM

The Cranial Nerves

Sometimes thought the most important nerves in the entire body, the cranial nerves all connect with the brain, keeping it directly in touch with the world outside. There are 12 pairs of these nerves. One nerve from each pair serves one side of the body, the other nerve supplies the other side.

Cranial nerves are still known by the numbering system supposedly introduced by Galen, a Greek doctor who died about AD200.

Our large diagram of the base of the brain shows that the cranial nerves start or end at the brain in an orderly sequence. Number 1 ends in bulbs below the front of the cerebrum. Number 2 ends in the cerebrum. Nerves 3 through 12 join parts of the brainstem thus: 3 and 4, the midbrain; 5 through 8, the pons; 9 through 12, the medulla. Dotted lines indicate sensory nerves; solid lines show motor nerves. Three nerves (1, 2 and 8) simply receive messages flowing into the brain. Two nerves (11 and 12) only send out signals to muscles. All the others both receive and transmit.

Three pairs of nerves (numbers 1, 2 and 8) feed the brain signals from those specialized sensory organs the nose, eyes and ears. Three more pairs (numbers 3, 4 and 6) supply the six muscles that work each eye. The fifth and seventh nerves are concerned with facial sensation and movement. The ninth, tenth, eleventh and twelfth cranial nerves between them handle sensation or movement in tongue, throat, shoulder, heart and abdominal organs.

Subsequent small diagrams show the parts of the body that each cranial nerve supplies.

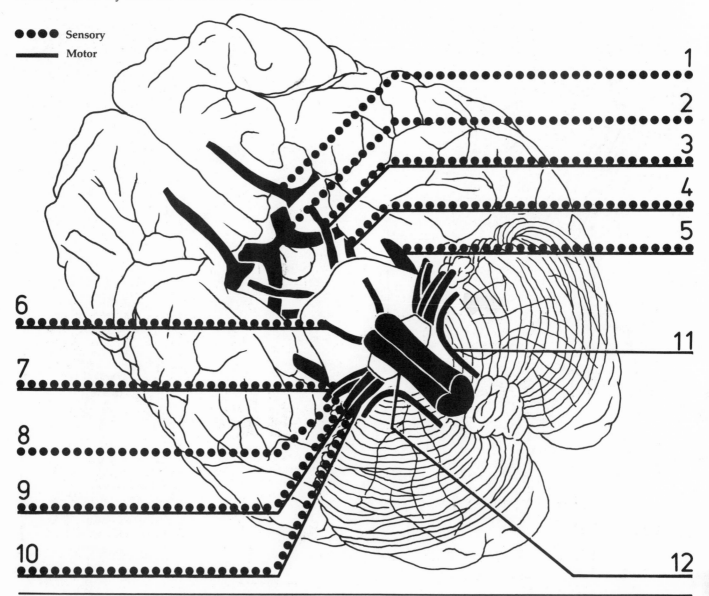

●●●● Sensory

———— Motor

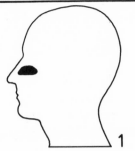

1 Olfactory Nerve
This feeds the brain "smell" signals from the mucous membrane high in the nostril. Smells may be classified as basically flowery, fruity, resinous, spicy, putrid and burnt.

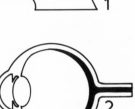

2 Optic Nerve
This sends to the brain signals produced when images appear on the retina at the back of the eye, and so makes sight possible.

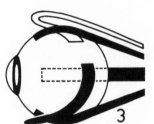

3 Oculomotor Nerve
This works four of the six muscles that move the eye, and the muscle that controls the size and reactions of the pupil.

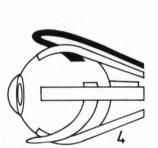

4 Trochlear Nerve
This nerve works the eye's superior oblique "pulley" muscle and coordinates with nerves 3 and 6.

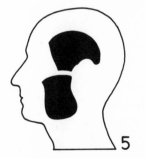

5 Trigeminal Nerve
This three-part nerve transmits sensations from the facial skin and from the eyes, nose, mouth and teeth (eg "runny" nose, dry eyes, toothache). It also tells the jaw muscles to chew.

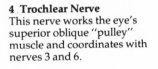

6 Abducens Nerve
This abducting nerve controls the outer muscle of the eye and coordinates with nerves 3 and 4.

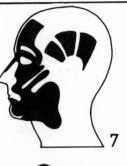

7 Facial Nerve
This nerve brings sensations of taste to the brain from the front of the tongue. But its main job is working the muscles that control facial expression – smiling, for example.

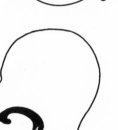

8 Acoustic Nerve
This sends sounds entering the ear to the brain as nerve impulses, so enabling you to hear. It also sends signals from the cochlea, a balance organ in the ear, telling the body if it is balanced or falling.

9 Glossopharyngeal Nerve
With part of the seventh nerve, this nerve sends the brain taste sensations. It also sends signals from the pharynx and helps to work the muscles needed for speech.

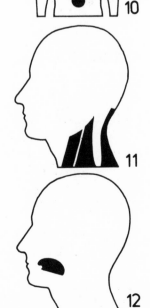

10 Vagus Nerve
This nerve supplies heart, lungs, stomach, kidneys and intestines. The vagus nerve automatically helps to regulate breathing, heartbeat and digestion.

11 Accessory Nerve
Also called the spinal accessory nerve, this cranial nerve sends to the muscles of the neck and back signals that turn the head and the shoulders.

12 Hypoglossal Nerve
This "under-tongue" twelfth cranial nerve carries motor signals from the brain to the tongue. Poking out the tongue and using the tongue in talking both involve this nerve.

©DIAGRAM

Nerves and Neurons

The billions of tiny active units making up the nervous system are neurons or nerve cells – cells designed to communicate electrochemically with one another. Several kinds of noncommunicating glial ("glue") cells support, nourish, insulate and far outnumber the neurons.

Each neuron receives and transmits signals through thousands of tiny "wires" linking it with other neurons in the nervous system. In fact these wires belong to the neurons themselves.

Each neuron has three main parts: cell body, axon and dendrites.

The cell body is a minute blob made up of a central nucleus surrounded by cytoplasm – a rather sticky fluid containing special microscopic structures. Nutrients and waste products filtering in and out through the permeable cell wall keep the cell body alive.

Thus far, neurons seem like the other cells that build our bodies. It is their projecting axons and dendrites that make them so remarkable.

An axon ("axis") is a long, slim "tree-trunk" transmitting signals from the cell body to other cells via junctions known as synapses. Axons linking nearby regions of nerve tissue may be no more than a few millimeters long, while others sending signals from remote parts of the body to the brain or vice versa can measure more than a yard (about 1m).

Dendrites ("like trees") are networks of short fibers that branch out from an axon and synapse with the ends of axons from other neurons. Dendrites are receivers, bringing signals to their neuron's own cell body.

Neurons come in many varieties, but all may be grouped in one of several ways, according to their purpose, size or shape. For instance, afferents (or sensory neurons) bring signals to the central nervous system from elsewhere in the body. Efferents (or motor neurons) send signals out. Interneurons – 97 per cent of all neurons, but found only in the brain and spinal cord – communicate between the other groups.

The gray matter of the brain and spinal cord consists of cell bodies. White matter comprises the nerve fibers, or axons, sheathed in a white fatty substance (myelin) which wraps around them in a roll. Bundles of such insulated axons form nerve fibers. Most central nervous system nerves comprise cell bodies with short axon tracts or bundles. The longest axons are in the peripheral nervous system. Outside the central nervous system, cell bodies clumped together form ganglia.

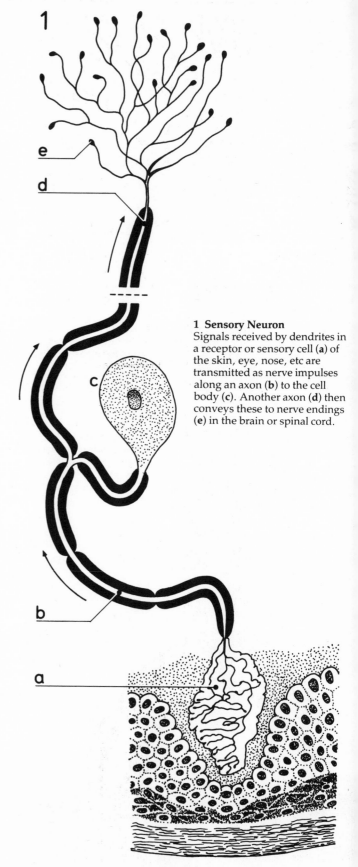

1 Sensory Neuron
Signals received by dendrites in a receptor or sensory cell (**a**) of the skin, eye, nose, etc are transmitted as nerve impulses along an axon (**b**) to the cell body (**c**). Another axon (**d**) then conveys these to nerve endings (**e**) in the brain or spinal cord.

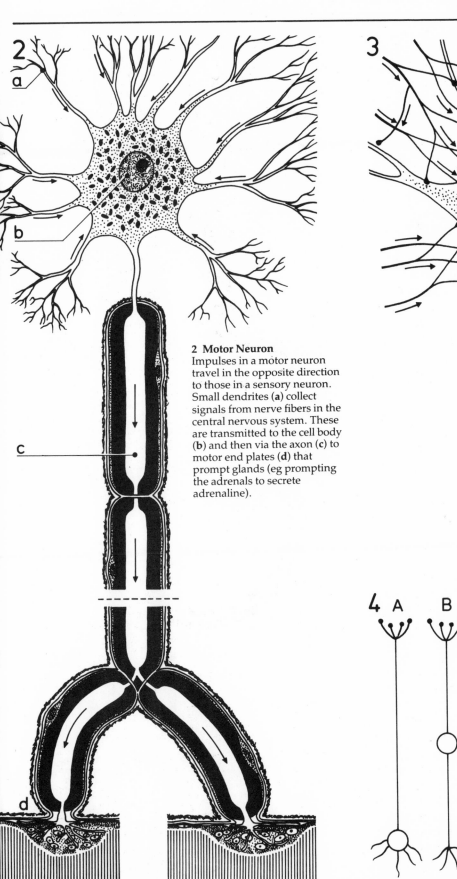

2 Motor Neuron
Impulses in a motor neuron travel in the opposite direction to those in a sensory neuron. Small dendrites (**a**) collect signals from nerve fibers in the central nervous system. These are transmitted to the cell body (**b**) and then via the axon (**c**) to motor end plates (**d**) that prompt glands (eg prompting the adrenals to secrete adrenaline).

3 Synaptic Contact
Neurons do not link directly with one another, but most neurons are indirectly linked with others via a synapse which enables impulses to pass between nerves. The cell body and dendrites of a typical motor neuron can have connections with hundreds, sometimes thousands, of other neurons. Note how small the synapses (**a**) are, compared with the cell body (**b**).

4 Types of Neuron
There are many different types of neuron of which only a few are shown here. They are often named with reference to the number of processes leading from the cell body.
A Multipolar neurons are the commonest sort and are found everywhere in the central nervous system.
B Bipolar neurons have a single process (dendron) leading into the cell body and a single process (axon) leaving it. They are mostly found in the retina.
C Pseudo-unipolar neurons are found in the chain of ganglia parallel with the spinal cord.

©DIAGRAM

Transmission of Information

Signals course through the nervous system in a relay where electrical impulses alternate with chemical messengers. The electrical impulses flow through those nerve-cell pathways the axons and dendrites. Chemical messengers leap the gaps (synapses) between each neuron's axon and the dendrites of the other neurons with which that axon makes contact. What happens is this. Before an impulse arrives, an inactive neuron has more potassium ions (electrically charged potassium atoms) than sodium ions. Outside the neuron the opposite holds good. So there are opposite electrical charges on the inside and the outside of the neuron's membrane.

When an impulse reaches the nearby axon tip of another neuron, this yields neurotransmitters. These chemicals burst from tiny sacs in the buttons forming the ends of the axon. Crossing the narrow synaptic gap between their axon and the inactive neuron's cell body or dendrites, the neurotransmitters lock onto receptor sites in the inactive neuron's cell membranes. This may let potassium ions out and sodium ions in, so altering the charge inside the membrane. Neurotransmitters like acetylcholine (in parts of the brain) and noradrenaline (in the brainstem and hypothalamus) make an electric impulse flow through the receiving neuron. Such chemicals are accordingly known as excitatory neurotransmitters.

But there are inhibitory neurotransmitters, too. Gamma amino butyric acid, or GABA, (in the brain's outer gray matter) and glycine (in the spinal cord) both act to block electrical impulses.

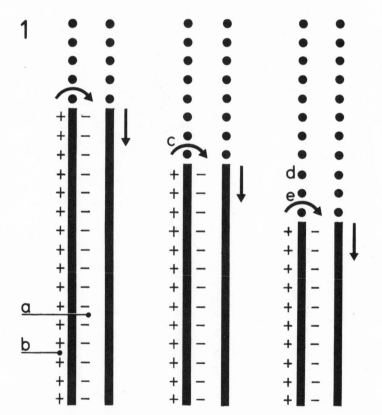

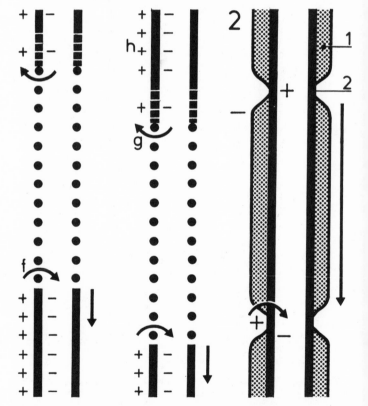

1 The Nerve Impulse
A nerve impulse is a wave of changing electric charge that passes down an axon from the cell body. A resting or unstimulated neuron has an active mechanism that keeps the inside of the cell (**a**) negatively charged and the area outside the cell membrane (**b**) positively charged. When a neuron is stimulated the permeability of the membrane alters, letting positively charged sodium ions flood into the cell (**c**). This briefly reverses the charge on either side of the membrane. This area of reversed charge (**d**) is the nerve impulse which excites an identical change in the area adjacent to it (**e**), this in turn activating the next area (**f**) and so on all the way down the axon. Once the nerve impulse has passed, sodium ions are pumped back out of the cell (**g**). After a brief recovery period the original charged state is restored (**h**) and the axon is ready to conduct another impulse.

2 Myelinated Neurons
Axons covered by a myelin sheath (**1**) conduct impulses up to twelve times faster than those without. Instead of a continuous wave moving down the axon, the impulse jumps between gaps in the sheath called nodes of Ranvier (**2**). Only in these areas does the charge become reversed.

At any instant, one brain cell may receive thousands of contradictory signals from the other cells with which it is in contact. Whether or not it fires off an electrical impulse depends on how many signals of each kind it receives. So neurons are really minute information processors, and their selective work prevents mental chaos.

Once a cell fires, the strength and speed of the impulse it carries depends on its dendrites and axon. The farther a signal flows through the dendrites, the weaker it grows. This is not true in axons, however long or short these may be. An axon's insulating myelin sheath may even boost the signal a little.

But axon size does affect axon speed. In the smallest axons, impulses crawl at a slothful 1mph (0.5m/sec). They zoom through the largest axons at 270mph (120m/sec). Yet even this rapid transit is considerably slower than an electric current flowing through a wire.

As electroencephalography shows, the brain is always firing with electrochemical activity. Yet, somehow, it sorts out for attention only those signals that matter. It can do this because a neuron's cell membrane can switch from negative to positive and back again in no more than one-thousandth of a second, and strongly stimulated neurons fire faster than others. Thus an excited neuron's 1000 firings per second stand out from the general background "noise" as a burst of machine-gun fire stands out from rifle shots.

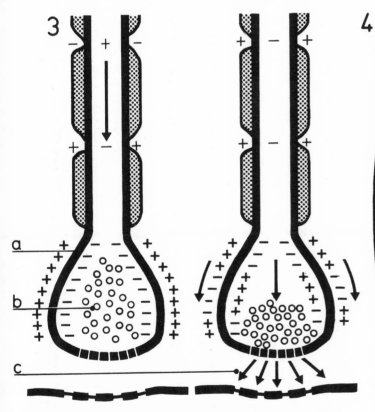

3 The Synapse
When a nerve impulse arrives at the membrane-covered synaptic button (**a**) at the end of an axon, it causes the tiny sacs (**b**) to fuse with the membrane and release a chemical neurotransmitter. This travels across the narrow gap (**c**) between one neuron and the next, triggering an impulse in the second neuron by making its membrane permeable to sodium ions.

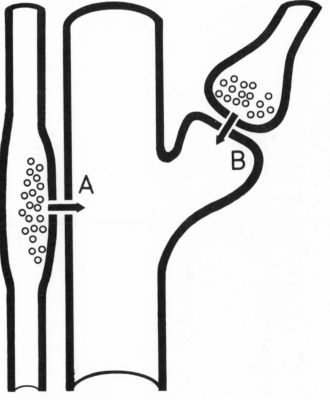

4 Types of Synapse
There are many variations on the simple synaptic contact. Contacts that occur between axons and dendrites that are side by side are known as parallel synapses (**A**). In other cases dendrites have small processes branching out from the side, and these form spinous or spiny synapses (**B**).

©DIAGRAM

Nerve Pathways

A brain cut open seems a meaningless mesh of neurons. Yet a signal speeding through the nervous system manages to find the exact region of the brain designed to handle it. Somehow, too, that region may send directions that reach specific muscles. All this is possible because the brain is built rather like a telephone exchange, with nerve fibers as its wiring and special neuron clusters as the switchboards controlling signals flowing in or out.

Special centers like the cerebral cortex or the cerebellum are relatively huge. Others, including some hidden in the brainstem, are cell clusters so small that you need a microscope to see them.

On close inspection, the maze of "wires" between these switchboards largely consists of ordered bundles of nerve fibers known as tracts. Each tract is made of axons projecting from cell bodies located in one "switchboard," and ending at one or more other "switchboards."

Hundreds of millions of these fibers supply different regions of the cerebrum. There are three main kinds of connection. Association fibers join different parts of the same cerebral hemisphere. Projection fibers fan out from the brainstem to all parts of the cerebrum. A dense mass of commissural fibers builds the corpus callosum – the bridge 4 inches (10cm) long that links both hemispheres.

Many fiber tracts are named according to where they start and finish. For example, corticospinal tract fibers send signals from cerebral cortex to spinal cord. Within such tracts, scientists have now discovered many pathways serving special purposes. Among others they have mapped the closely associated pain and temperature pathways, and the general sensory pathways.

From such studies we now know that different spinal nerves serve specific regions of the body surface, known as dermatones. This helps explain why disorder of an internal organ that affects a spinal nerve may produce pain that seems located in the skin some way from the actual trouble. This phenomenon is called referred pain and may result, for example, in gallbladder pain being felt in the right shoulder.

Even when a pathway has been severed, its central nervous system "switchboard" may report incoming calls. Thus certain stimuli produce "phantom limb" sensation in amputees. Some actually claim to sense a wristwatch on a missing arm.

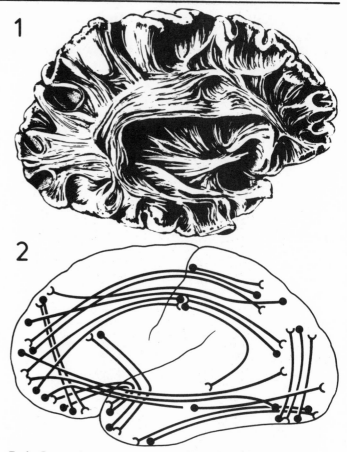

Brain Connections
The brain is much more complicated than any diagram can show; thousands of nerve tracts can be seen in the vertical cross-section (1) and millions more are visible when the brain is examined under the microscope. The diagram (2) shows a few of the association fibers that connect different areas of the same cerebral hemisphere. The horizontal cross-section (3) shows how corresponding areas in the cerebral hemispheres on opposite sides of the brain are connected by nerve tracts that pass through the central corpus callosum bridge.

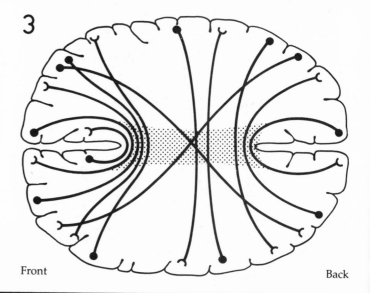

Front   Back

4 Nerve pathways
Most activities require many different parts of the brain to work together. The dotted lines show a sensory nerve carrying an impulse from a touch receptor (**a**) in the skin into the spinal cord (**b**), from where it reaches five different brain areas – the cerebellum (**c**), concerned with fine control of movement; the corpora quadrigemina (**d**) in the brainstem; the thalamus (**e**) in the midbrain; the hypothalamus (**f**); and the cerebral cortex (**g**) where conscious thought originates and the touch sensation is interpreted. The solid lines show that to move a muscle (**h**), a command comes from the cerebral cortex but extra information is fed into the motor nerve from one of the same areas (**c**) that initially interpreted the touch impulse.

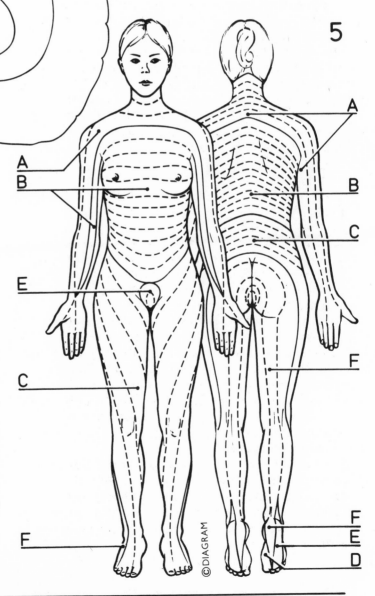

5 Dermatones
The body's surface is really a collection of distinct areas (dermatones), each supplied by a different spinal nerve. The dotted lines show the boundaries between one dermatone and the next and the solid lines represent the boundaries between the groups of dermatones supplied by the set of nerves from one part of the spinal cord. Area **A** is supplied by the cervical nerves; **B** – the chest and part of the arm – by thoracic nerves; **C** and **D** by lumbar nerves; **E** and **F** by sacral nerves. Pain in a dermatone may be the result of something wrong with the internal organ supplied by the same nerve that supplies the dermatone. The pain of a heart attack, for example, is often felt in the left arm, which is supplied by the set of thoracic nerves that supplies the heart.

Chapter 3

DEVELOPMENT OF THE BRAIN

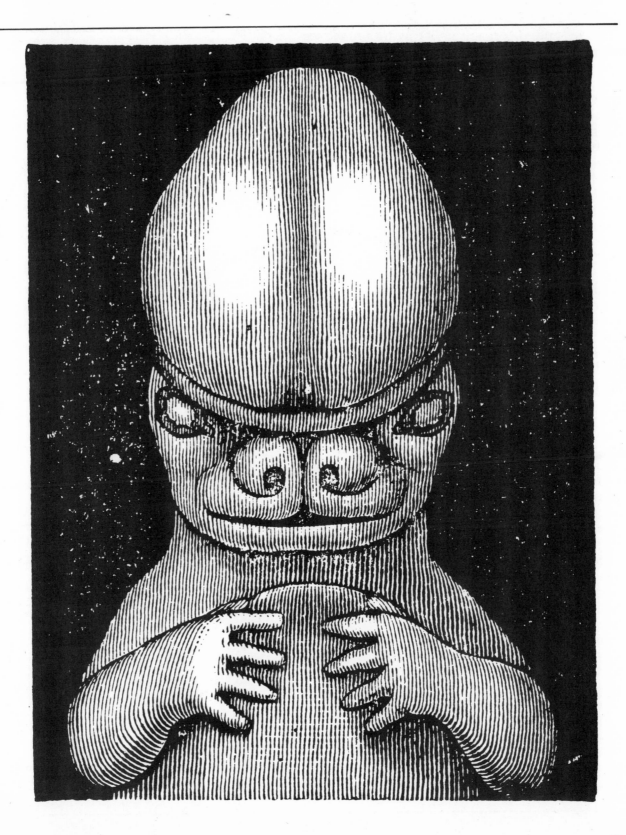

The Evolving Brain

Our multi-million nerve-cell central nervous system has its evolutionary roots in the scattered nerve cells of tiny, lowly organisms that lived in water more than 500 million years ago. Nerve cells evidently first appeared in coelenterates – "hollow-gutted" organisms like hydra and the sea-anemone. A coelenterate's nerve network lacks any kind of centralized control. This probably began with flatworms – the first creatures to possess a head. Specialized sense cells help flatworms respond more flexibly than sea anemones to outside stimuli. But like most animals without a backbone, flatworms act mostly by instinct and reflex.

Intelligent behavior remained impossible until the evolution of relatively big, complex types of brain – the types we find among the backboned animals, or vertebrates. The tiniest fish has a larger brain than the largest insect. But the development of a fish's three-part brain reflects that beast's unintellectual priorities. Much of the forebrain deals only with smell. The midbrain handles vision, the hindbrain, balance.

From fishes came amphibians, which gave rise in their turn to reptiles – creatures with a type of brain evolved for land-based life. The reptile's enlarged midbrain and hindbrain accompany improved vision and hearing and the midbrain's increased role as a coordinator of sensory activities.

With early mammals the brain grew larger and more complex. Sense coordination shifted from the midbrain to the forebrain, an evolving structure capped by a folded cerebrum to handle memory and learning. Meanwhile the hindbrain gained a large cerebellum to coordinate complicated movements.

Advanced mammals such as monkeys, apes and man (the primates) have brains derived from ancestors that took to living in the trees, where vision mattered more than smell. Accordingly the once-big "smell" part of the forebrain devolved, while the part that handles vision grew much larger.

This helped to trigger an enormous growth in brain size and complexity, especially in man, whose nimble fingers, upright stance and capacity for speech opened up new opportunities for hand-eye coordination and scope for abstract thought – a faculty located in the cerebral cortex.

In us, then, that once tiny outgrowth of the forebrain now dwarfs and dominates both midbrain and hindbrain, and its evolution has totally remodeled the conformation of the skull.

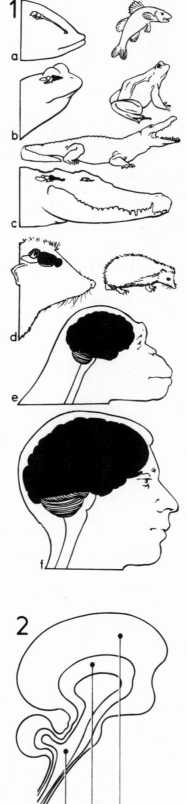

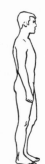

1 Vertebrate Brains
Brains of six living backboned animals mirror stages in the evolution of the brain from prehistoric fish to man. In the frog and crocodile, the forebrain (shaded) seems mostly taken up by the olfactory bulb – concerned with smell. In a hedgehog the forebrain covers the front end of the brainstem. In a chimpanzee and man the forebrain's cerebrum has overgrown almost all the more primitive structures of the brain.
a Fish.
b Frog (amphibian).
c Crocodile (reptile).
d Hedgehog (mammal).
e Chimpanzee (mammal).
f Man (mammal).

2 Our Layered Brain
The American scientist Paul MacLean has argued that man's brain has three layers that betray its evolutionary past as layered rocks reveal the story of the Earth's crust. He called these layers reptilian (A); paleomammalian or "old mammalian" (B); neomammalian or "new mammalian" (C). According to this notion, the reptilian brain in hindbrain and midbrain is a slave to precedent; the paleomammalian brain around the top of the brainstem, the seat of the emotions; and reason resides only in the neomammalian brain or cerebral cortex. Some experts find MacLean's interpretation oversimple.

3 Increasing Brain Size
Anthropologists studying the
brain capacity of past and
present skulls show that man's
brain has grown relatively and
absolutely larger since his early
ancestors roamed Africa more
than two million years ago.
Cubes (right) show cubic
capacity of past and present
brains of human type, with a
prediction for "tomorrow's
man."
a *Australopithecus* (southern
ape): 450cc, about 5 million
years ago. This African man-
ape may not have been one of
our direct ancestors.
b *Homo* 1470: 800cc, about 2.5
million years ago. Such
hominids may have led directly
to men of modern type.
c *Homo erectus* (upright man):
1000cc, 1.5 million years ago.
d *Homo erectus* (a later
subspecies): 1200cc, 500,000
years ago.
e *Homo sapiens* (wise man):
1400cc, 50,000 years ago to
today. Brain size has remained
about the same since late Old
Stone Age times.
f Tomorrow's man: selective
breeding, perhaps boosted by
genetic engineering, could
theoretically produce men with
bigger, wiser brains than any
now alive.

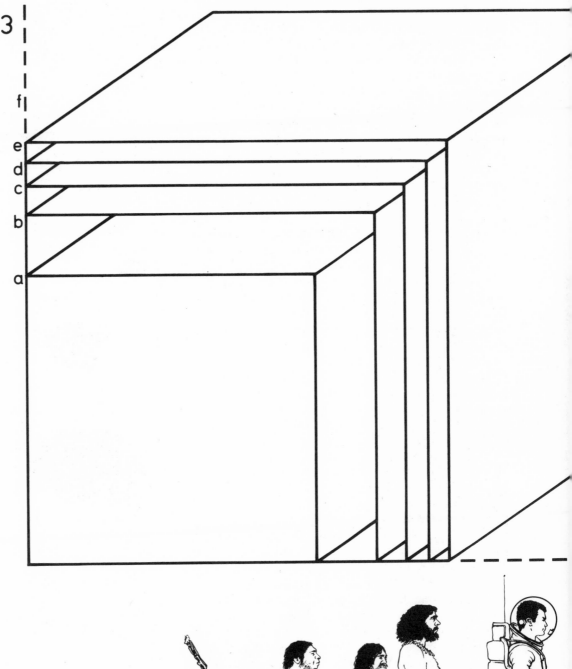

4 Primate Brains
Brain developments matched
changing modes of life among
evolving primates.
a Keen-eyed prosimians lived
in trees 60 million years ago.
b Man's pre-ape ancestor
moved on all fours 40 million
years ago.
c *Ramapithecus* could walk on
hind legs and brandish sticks,
14 million years ago.
d *Australopithecus* probably
used sharp stones as tools, 5
million years ago.
e *Homo* 1470 sharpened stones
(the first true tools?) 2.5 million
years ago.
f *Homo erectus* had learned to
use fire 500,000 years ago.
g *Homo sapiens* had complex
tool kits by 40,000 years ago.

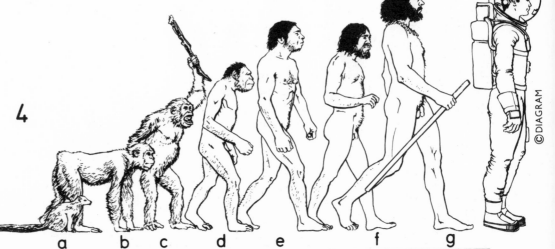

©DIAGRAM

The Growing Brain

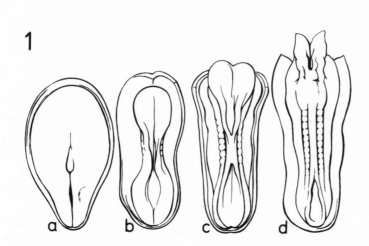

1

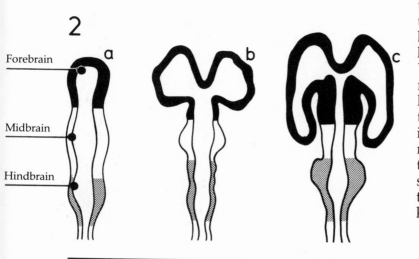

1 The Budding Brain
A back view of a human embryo shows how the spinal cord and brain begin to grow.
a A six-day-old embryo shows few signs of brain or cord.
b By 20 days an outer layer of cells throws up parallel waves separated by a groove.
c By 22 days, wave crests are meeting to form a neural tube – basic structure for the spinal cord and brain.
d At 23 days the embryo has paired structures bulging from the front (here top) end of the neural tube. These are the beginnings of the brain. Failure of the front end of the neural groove to close results in anencephaly (an undeveloped brain).

2 The Three-Part Brain
Enlarged sections along an embryonic brain show stages in the development of its three main regions.
a Only 25 days following conception the embryonic brain has three main vesicles, foreshadowing division into forebrain, midbrain, hindbrain.
b The three vesicles have become five. The hollow that they enclose will later give rise to ventricles – cavities within the brain. The forebrain now grows rapidly.
c Later still, the bulging forebrain contains the makings of cerebral hemispheres and inner structures. The bulge below the midbrain includes the budding cerebellum.

Forebrain

Midbrain

Hindbrain

Brain growth during development inside the womb and in the five years after birth proceeds astonishingly fast, compared with growth in other parts of the body.

The first signs of the brain appear in an embryo only three weeks or so after conception, when the embryo is only 3mm long. Its budding brain starts as a swelling at one end of the so-called neural tube formed by waves of tissue that rise and fuse along what becomes the curved back of the embryo. Major regions of the human brain develop in a sequence reminiscent of its evolution. The brainstem develops first. But by five weeks all three main regions are recognizable, the forebrain twisted sharply downward. By 10 weeks the forebrain's cerebral hemispheres have outgrown other regions, and begun to overlap the brainstem. That "little brain" the cerebellum starts its growth spurt somewhat later.

This prebirth increase in size results from cells multiplying in the brain. In 1970 British researchers John Dobbing and Jean Sands discovered two main phases when brain cells are multiplying very rapidly. Their research results showed cells proliferating quickly in 15–20-week-old fetuses. The team judged this coincided with a spurt in neuron output. At 25 weeks another spurt began, persisting less intensively to birth and for a year beyond. Dobbing and Sands surmised this coincided with the growth of glial ("glue") cells, not of yet more neurons.

Collectively, the brain and other parts of the nervous system grow faster before birth and in the early years of life than muscles, genitals or other body components. This is why a two-month fetal head is almost half body length. Indeed a newborn baby's brain has reached one quarter of its adult weight already, although the baby is only one-twentieth as heavy as the adult it will become. In the next six months a child's brain weight doubles. By the age of 5 or so, its brain is nine-tenths as heavy as it will ever be.

Yet though the newborn baby has almost all the neurons (nerve cells) its brain will ever hold, they have yet to form a subtle mesh of links – the mesh that helps transform this kit of parts into a fully integrated mechanism. Scientists used to think neurons linked up haphazardly. Now they believe the nervous system includes chemically coded specifications determining where neurons latch on to one another. The forging of these links holds a key to the maturing of the brain.

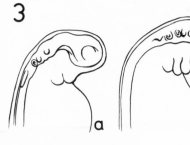

3

a b c d e

3 The Brain Takes Shape

Here we show nine stages in brain growth as an embryo becomes a fetus and this grows into a newborn infant. These illustrations reveal that the most dramatic developments happen in the first few weeks as the head takes shape, largely to accommodate the fast-bulging forebrain.

a A three-week-old embryo's emergent brain somewhat resembles the knobbly handle of a miniature walking stick.

b By four weeks the forebrain is already swelling and curving downward.

c At five weeks you can plainly see an eye bud growing from this forebrain (the retina in a fully formed eye is a budded-off extension of the brain). Farther back toward the spinal cord, the cranial nerves are sprouting from the future brainstem.

d At seven weeks these developments show further progress. Now, too, a deep crease in the forebrain behind the budding eye hints at the forebrain's division into telencephalon ("endbrain")

where outpocketings will become the left and right cerebral hemispheres, and diencephalon ("between brain") where the hypothalamus and thalamus take shape.

e At 11 weeks, telencephalon has overlapped diencephalon and a narrow "scarf" around the brainstem shows the emergent cerebellum. From now on the telencephalon and cerebellum are the major areas of growth.

f At four months telencephalon and cerebellum have met: the optic nerve is well developed and the lateral cerebral fissure has formed as a deep groove in the side of the brain.

g By six months grooves and ridges are appearing in the expanding telencephalon.

h By eight months grooves and ridges are pronounced.

i This newborn baby's telencephalon is deeply wrinkled to maximize the cerebral surface area that can be crammed inside its skull.

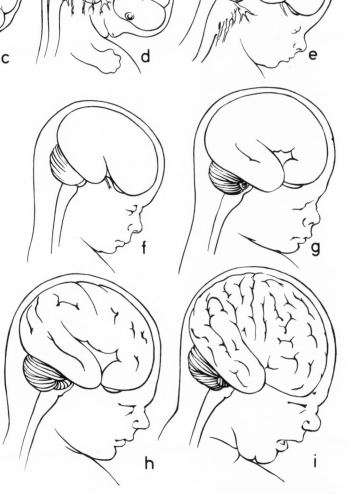

f g h i

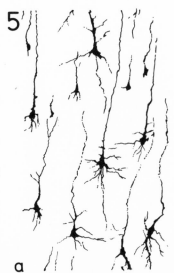

4

Man	Chimp	100%
	65%	
		50%
25%		

4 Brain Size at Birth

Here we show brain sizes of man and chimpanzee at birth as percentages of adult brain size. A young chimpanzee's well-developed brain gives it early learning advantages, but its precocity is soon outstripped by the rapid growth of the human offspring's brain.

5 How Nerves Grow

Neurons in a language center of the brain are simple and well spaced at birth (**a**). By six years old (**b**) they have grown many interconnections. Chemical codes incorporated in the brain seemingly decide exactly how and where such pathways will develop.

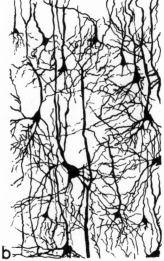

5

a b

©DIAGRAM

Development of Motor Control

Motor control advances in a sequence affected by the order of development of different regions of the brain and the rest of the nervous system. Key factors include the growth of pathways between individual neurons, and the growth of insulating myelin sheaths, which help to convey the signals that course through many neurons. Fine muscle control depends on the maturation of such special brain areas as the cerebellum, which helps to check unwanted muscle movements.

Children control central body areas (eg upper arms and legs) before outer areas. Control also follows a head-to-foot sequence, eg head-lifting, body-hauling, then crawling. Lastly, control works from big to small muscles. Thus walking practice is useless until the brain is ready for it.

1 Primitive Reflexes
Newborn babies respond to certain stimuli by reflex movements – a legacy from the remote past when the nervous system worked mostly at an instinctive level.
a Rooting reflex. A baby turns its nipple-seeking mouth toward a touch on the cheek.
b Asymmetric tonic neck reflex. This is the position adopted by a newborn baby lying on its back.
c Grasp reflex.
d Crossed extension reflex. Stroking an extended foot makes the other leg react.
e Moro (startle) reflex.
f Walking reflex. The baby cannot truly walk of course.
g Stepping reflex.

2 Secondary Responses
These reflexes appear as primitive reflexes decline, at about four months. Some may come later. They involve balancing, rolling, and protecting the falling body.
a Downward parachute. A swiftly lowered baby stretches his legs ready for landing.
b Forward parachute. A baby tilted forward protectively extends his arms and fingers.
c Rolling response. Rolled over by his legs, the baby responds with automatic head and arm movements.
d Sideways propping reaction. If a sitting child is tilted sideways he extends an arm and hand, pressing down to stop his body falling.

3 Motor Landmarks
Right-hand illustrations show the first 13 months' progress in motor control, mirroring the brain's developing ability to control muscles used in sitting, walking, crawling and grasping.
a This is the flaccid posture of a newborn baby held to sit.
b Held to sit at four weeks, a baby briefly lifts his head.
c By 12 weeks a supported baby holds his head up.
d By 20 weeks the seated baby keeps a straight back.
e At 28 weeks he can sit alone supported by his arms.
f At 36 weeks he can adjust his balance by bending his body forward.
g By 48 weeks he can twist around to pick something up, yet also keep his balance.

h A newborn baby held like this performs purely reflex walking actions.
i Held in a standing posture, the eight-week baby briefly keeps his head up.
j The 36-week old can stand by grasping furniture.
k At 48 weeks a child can walk if his hands are held.
l The 13-month-old child can walk unaided.

m Laid prone, a newborn baby draws knees beneath abdomen.
n The six-week baby lies less tucked up, and turns his head to the side.
o At 12 weeks the baby lies extended and may lift his chin and shoulders.
p By 20 weeks the prone baby raises head and upper chest.
q By 24 weeks he raises head, chest and upper abdomen.
r The 36-week old finds he can go backward by pushing down and forward on a surface.
s By 44 weeks he coordinates arms and legs to crawl forward on hands and knees.

t The newborn's fingers clutch with reflex grip.
u The six-month child can deliberately grasp a cube.
v By eight months he grips with thumb opposite fingers.
w By nine months thumb and finger grip are more precise.
x By one year old thumb and finger grip are mature.
As the cerebellum learns to control "automatic" acts, other brain regions are freed for simultaneous but different activities.

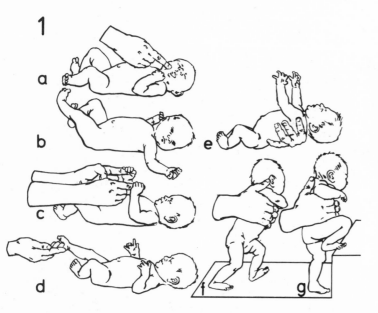

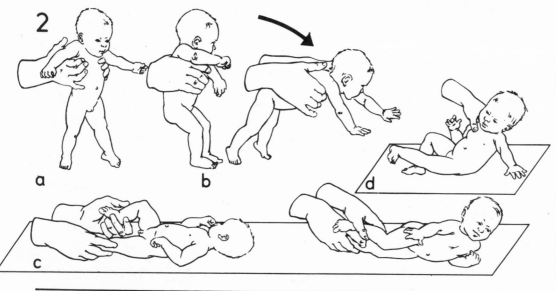

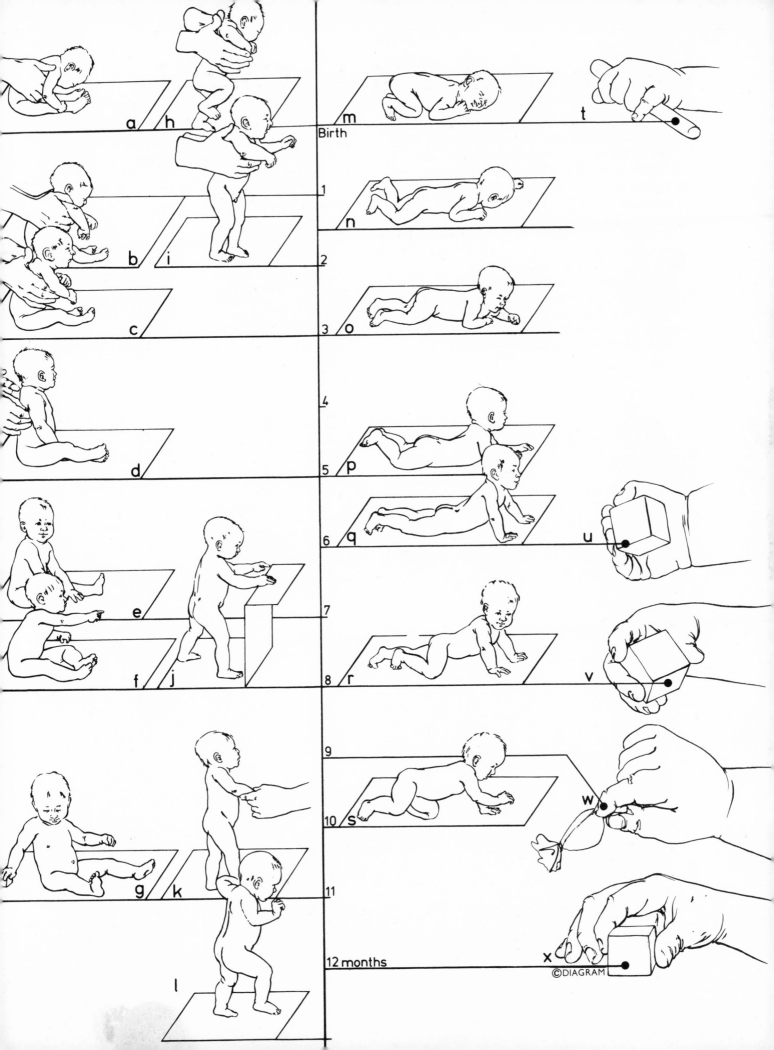

a h

Birth

m t

b i

1

n

c

2

3 o

d

4

5 p

e j

6 q u

7

f r v

8

9

g k

10 s w

11

l

12 months x

©DIAGRAM

Development of Sight and Speech

Basic mechanisms for sight, hearing and making vocal sounds are built into the brain by birth. Experiments with newborn kittens reveal visual detectors already formed inside the brain. Tests with newborn infants show eyes try to find and fixate big black dots on a white strip being drawn by motor above the baby's head. This is just a reflex action, and young babies cannot see as well as we do. The eyes' retinas are not properly developed and nerves coursing from the eyes through the brain still lack insulating sheaths of myelin. But eye-brain development soon gets good enough for pattern recognition. By two weeks some babies spend more time looking at a face-like pattern than at one with the same elements randomly arranged. They are learning to perceive.

Astonishing experiments with kittens and young monkeys have revealed a so-called sensitive period for the development of vision. Deprived of visual stimuli for just four days in its second month a kitten may be permanently blinded: brain cells registering signals from the eyes stop working and cannot be reactivated later. Similarly, young babies reach a critical phase when eye-use is essential to reconfirm existing visual ability.

There is also a critical period beyond which speech cannot be learned. Children reportedly brought up by wolves never master speech. Deaf children given hearing aids after one year old may suffer similarly. Uncommitted at birth, speech centers in the brain must be stimulated early if a baby is to learn to talk.

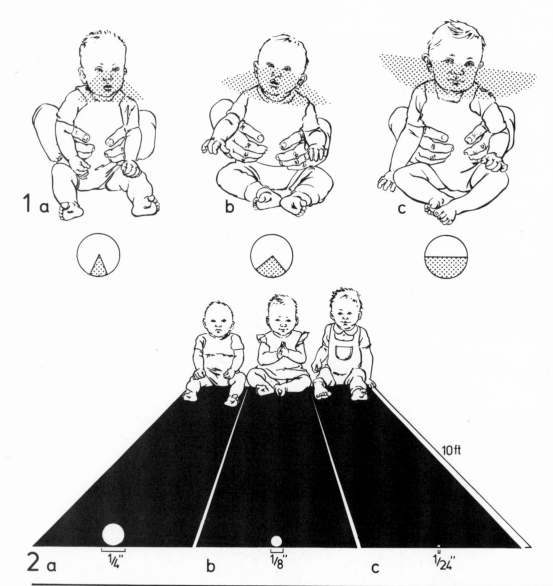

1 Field of Vision
At birth a baby's eyes move independently. He finds it hard to gaze on any object. Brain control of eye muscles contributes to improvements.
a Soon after birth he can watch a dangling ball swung through 45° – one-quarter of an adult's field of vision.
b By six weeks he moves his eyes to watch a ball through 90°. This coincides with the development of binocular vision. Both eyes can now focus on one object. Both send signals that converge to stimulate the same neurons at the back of the brain.
c By three months he has the full adult field of vision.

2 Depth of Vision
Tests with moving balls of differing diameters show how depth of vision improves in the first year. A month-old baby gazes at a small white ball 6–10in (15–25cm) away but not at one across a room.
a A six-month baby watches a ball ¼in (6mm) in diameter 10ft (3m) away. This implies visual acuity of 20/120 – ie ability clearly to focus an object 20ft away that someone with normal 20/20 vision sees clearly from 120ft.
b A nine-month baby watches a ball ⅛in (3mm) in diameter 10ft away. This implies 20/60 vision.
c At one year he has 20/20 (normal) visual acuity.

3 Development of Hearing

The hearing mechanism is fully formed at birth. A newborn baby reacts to harsh, sharp sounds. A 10-day baby responds to a voice or loudly ticking watch and soon responds to sounds differing in pitch and loudness. Sound localization improves over the first year, helped by improving coordination.

a The three-month baby turns vaguely toward a sound.
b The five-month baby turns, then inclines the head, to find a sound below ear level.
c By eight months turning and inclination begin merging.
d By nine to ten months the child swivels his head in a direct diagonal movement.

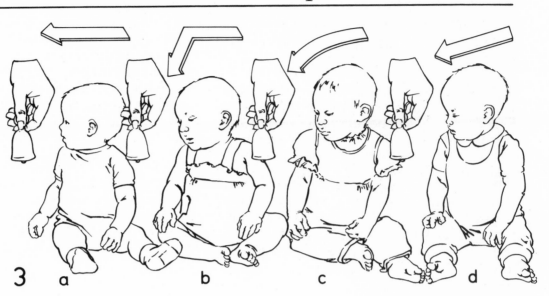

4 Sounds of Speech

Infants first learn to babble. Adults' responses teach them to select sounds they hear other people use. The order of appearance of speech sounds (phonemes) tends to follow a pattern. Children master easy or often-heard phonemes first. Complete mastery is not established until five to seven years.

A In an English-speaking land an eight-week child utters an "a" and some of the other vowel sounds.
M By 16 weeks he mouths "m," also "b," "g," "k," "p."
T By 32 weeks he can say "t," "d," "w."
S The sounds "s," "f," "h," "r," and "th" come later.

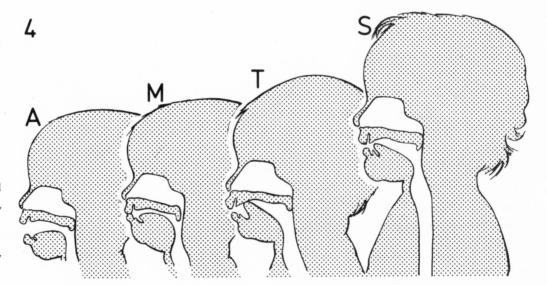

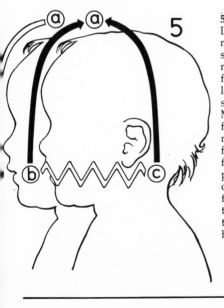

5 Learning to Speak

Learning to speak involves making and monitoring sounds. Speech occurs when motor nerves bearing signals from the brain (**a**) operate larynx, vocal cords, pharynx, soft palate, tongue and lips. Monitoring speech involves feedback to the brain. Sensory nerves bring the brain signals from speech muscles (**b**) and from the ears (**c**) which have picked up sound waves pushed out by the voice. Thanks to this feedback system, a child learns to modify the sounds he makes to match the words that he has heard other people speaking.

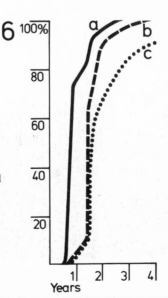

6 Speech Development

Speech development usually starts with vocalized vowels at about seven weeks. By 16 weeks a child utters some consonants. By 20 weeks he says some syllables. The first meaningful word usually appears by 44–48 weeks. By 21–24 months a child is using two-word phrases. By three years he talks incessantly. Our graph shows progress of speech development in tested groups of normal children from birth to four years old.

a Percentage uttering words.
b Percentage saying phrases.
c Percentage capable of intelligible speech.

©DIAGRAM

Conceptual Development

As children's brains mature they pass through several intellectual stages. At first they can only grapple with the here and now, and their brains' emotional and rational divisions overlap. Only as they reach their teens can they cope confidently with all kinds of abstract problems.

Experiments with laboratory animals suggest that normal intellectual development depends at least partly on environment. Stimulated rats grow brains with a thicker cerebral cortex, more glial cells, bigger neuron cell bodies, and more of certain neurotransmitters than rats reared in boredom. Thus understimulated children may have physically underdeveloped brains. Also, children malnourished in the womb or before 18 months of age can be intellectually impaired for life.

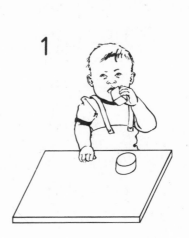

1 Visual Perception
For sighted people conceptual development is much helped by visual perception – the brain's chief source of information about the outside world. To newborn infants this world is a muddle of blotches. But perception of color, size and shape begin early. Three-month-old infants gaze longer at colored than at gray paper, for cones developed in the eye's retina now make color vision possible. At six months children reach for a small nearby rattle, not a larger one farther away, even though it looks as big. Also, they learn to recognize a sweetened square offered with other simple shapes.

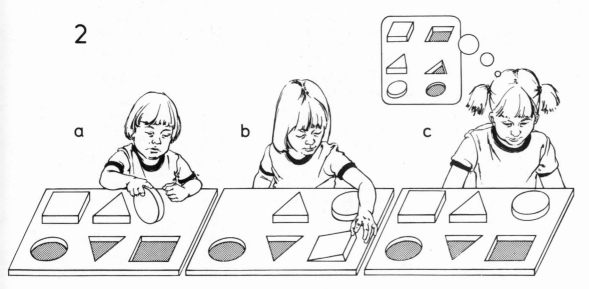

2 How Children Learn
A child tackles a form-board puzzle in different ways at different ages.
a At age two she tries forcing a block into a hole irrespective of their shapes.
b At 2½ if the block does not fit one hole she tries to push it into another.
c By age three she matches shapes by eye before acting. Language helps this process. Such tests suggest trial-and-error learning. The puzzle is a stimulus evoking a response of effort pleasurably rewarded by solving the puzzle. Thus effort and reward become associated in the brain. Next time the puzzle is presented, she will complete it faster.

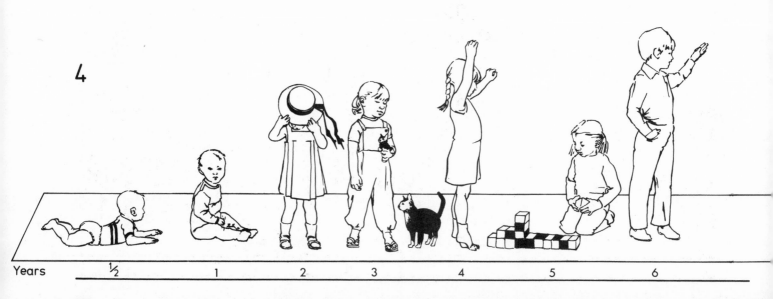

Years ½ 1 2 3 4 5 6

3 Piaget's Theories

The influential Swiss psychologist Jean Piaget said intellectual development goes through stages where cognition ("the act of knowing") and emotion interact.

1 Sensorimotor stage (0–2 years). Intelligence is empirical and largely non-verbal. Muscles and senses help children deal with external objects and events. They experiment with objects and graft new experience on old. They grasp that objects persist out of sight and touch. They start to symbolize – using words and gestures.

2 Preoperational stage (2–7 years). Children use words for perceived objects and inner feelings, and experimentally manipulate them in the mind. They act by trial and error, intuition and experience.

3 Concrete-operational stage (7–12 years). Logical operations begin. Children classify objects by similarities and differences.

4 Formal operations (12 years onward). Children use thought more flexibly, to handle hypothetical issues. Grasping conservation of amount and number are major landmarks. Before seven, a child seeing equal amounts of water poured into containers of unequal height may say a tall, narrow container (**a**) receives more water than a short, broad container (**b**).

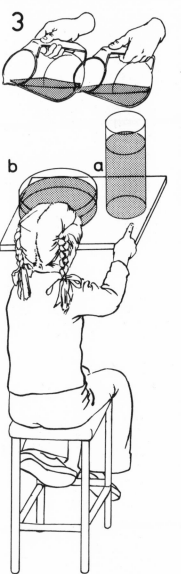

4 Stages in Development

Their maturing brains take children through stages of intellectual development. The following items give likely mental capabilities of children aged as shown below.

6 months Recognizes familiar faces. May perceive differences between some shapes.

1 year Says first words. Defines some objects by use.

1–2 years Manipulates objects in trial-and-error fashion. May use observation of cause and effect to solve some simple, practical problems by action.

2 Gives own first name. Knows difference between "one" and "many." Understands simple language.

2½ Knows many more words than he uses. Knows own sex.

2–4 Uses signs and symbols (words) to stand for absent objects and events but often confuses sign or symbol with the thing signified or symbolized. Thinks changing an object's shape alters its size, weight and volume.

3 Knows own age in years. Is gaining accurate visual judgment of depth. Knows the difference between "big" and "little."

4 Speaks fully intelligibly and uses many words. Knows "yesterday," "today," and "tomorrow." In reasoning often confuses cause and effect. Understands "higher," "longer" and "heavier."

4–7 Intelligent behavior largely limited to actions and intuitive thought based on incomplete perceptions.

5 Perceives relative sizes of objects well. Counts up to 15 bricks. May be learning to read. Can write some letters.

5–8 Intersensory perception developing rapidly.

6 May be learning to write joined-up letters by now. Can say days of the week. Counts up to 30 by rote. Knows "right" and "left."

7 Tells time from clock. Knows own birthday. Knows changing an object's shape need not change its size.

8 Reasons well about data he can see and touch. Solves simple mathematical problems. Enjoys reading children's books with more text than pictures.

8–11 Groups objects in classes and series. Fully grasps concepts of space, time and number.

9 Develops abstract response to the concept of weight.

10 Mental problem-solving improves.

11 Reasons logically about statements, not just about concrete objects and events.

12 Develops historical time sense. Is now well able to formulate hypotheses, make assumptions, and draw conclusions. Ability to reason increases through teens.

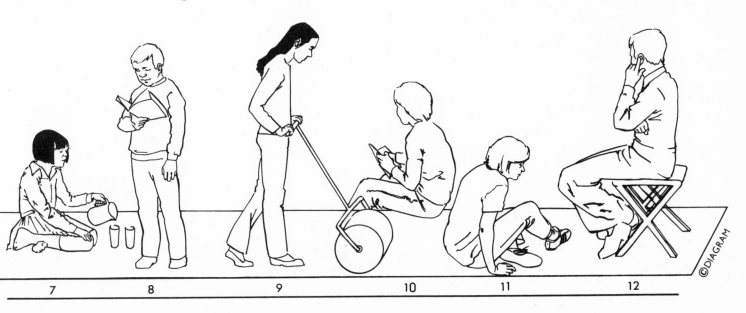

7   8   9   10   11   12

The Decline with Age

At birth our bodies come complete with all the nerve cells they will ever hold. This makes the brain unlike every other organ but the heart. In other organs, new cells grow to replace those that die. No new cells take the place of brain cells that wear out. By the time we reach the age of 20, brain cells are dying in their thousands every day. From then on our brains shrink as they lose weight by about 1 gram per year.

Old people's brains show measurable changes. The fissures of the brain are broad and deep; the ventricles – those natural cavities in the brain – have enlarged. Many of the surviving nerve cells are degenerating, often in the cerebellum and maybe other special regions of the brain. An additional reason for brain atrophy is narrowing of arteries. This reduces the brain's supply of vital oxygen and nutrients, and makes removing wastes less efficient.

The brain's slow physical decline goes hand in hand with a falling off in intellectual performance. At first this is too slight to show up in ordinary life. However, special intelligence tests reveal subtle changes under way from age 20 onward. One set of tests of so-called primary mental abilities shows marked changes in the over 50s. This age group reveals its greatest falling off in logical reasoning (solving rational problems – an ability that calls for planning, deduction and also generalizing from experience). Spatial reasoning (being able to consider objects in two or three dimensions) is hard hit too. Number ability (handling figures mentally) and verbal meaning (grasping verbally expressed ideas) stand up better to the aging

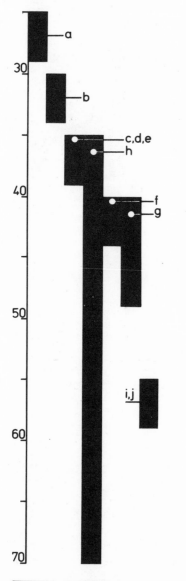

1 Age and Output
Studies of creative work produced by people outstanding in various fields show that peak periods of productivity occur before aging blunts the intellectual process. These examples (**a-h**) contrast with the main age groups (**i-j**) for successful politicians.

Creative people	Ages
a Poets	25–29
b Chemists	30–34
c Philosophers	35–39
d Playwrights	35–39
e Psychologists	35–39
f Best-selling novelists	40–44
g Metaphysicians	40–49
h American composers in the early 1900s	35–70
Politicians	
i American presidents	55–59
j Members of the British cabinet	55–59

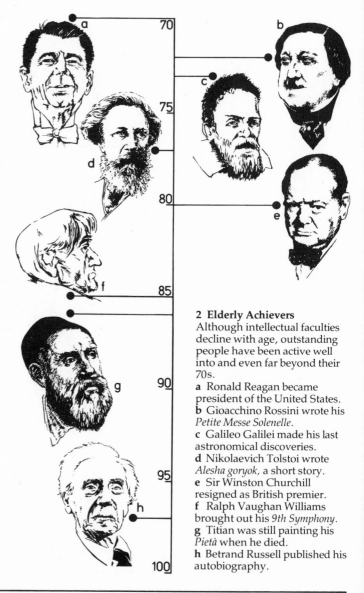

2 Elderly Achievers
Although intellectual faculties decline with age, outstanding people have been active well into and even far beyond their 70s.
a Ronald Reagan became president of the United States.
b Gioacchino Rossini wrote his *Petite Messe Solenelle.*
c Galileo Galilei made his last astronomical discoveries.
d Nikolaevich Tolstoi wrote *Alesha goryok,* a short story.
e Sir Winston Churchill resigned as British premier.
f Ralph Vaughan Williams brought out his *9th Symphony.*
g Titian was still painting his *Pietà* when he died.
h Betrand Russell published his autobiography.

process. But all such mental operations take longer than they used to.

The senses also suffer. Vision, hearing, taste and smell grow less efficient. Aging people perceive touch, movement and vibration less well than the young. Posture awareness and sense of balance are affected. Some nerve impulses slow down and the body's "thermostat" grows less effective at controlling body temperature.

However, increasing age brings some advantages. Accumulated experience helps to compensate for diminishing intelligence. Middle age, of course, is when many people reach the peak of their career, enjoying higher incomes and more social prestige than younger individuals still with much to learn.

Indeed, many leading statesmen are actually old, handling their responsibilities with wisdom based on decades of experience denied to younger people whose intellectual capacity is actually greater.

By the 70s the declining powers of the brain and senses may affect everyday activities. Impaired perception, slowed reactions, poor short-term memory, defective sight and hearing, and an unreliable sense of balance combine to make old people liable to accidents in street and home. Mental illness grows more likely in old age. The "thoughtless" behavior of some old people may reflect decay of the brain's higher centers. But many doctors see senile dementia as a disease, not part of the normal aging process. Then, too, "senile" behavior is sometimes due to treatable disease like myxedema. Most people remain mentally normal even in extreme old age.

3 Waning Intelligence

Graphs show how various components of intelligence vary with age as measured on the Wechsler-Bellevue scale (other tests give slightly different findings, but agree that intellectual capacity – though not attainment – peaks around the age of 20).

a Vocabulary: the ability to define words in a list.

b Information: remembering general knowledge facts.

c Comprehension: showing commonsense understanding.

d Arithmetic: handling simple numerical data.

e Similarities: discovering abstract relationships in separate subjects.

f Picture completion: spotting omissions in pictures of familiar objects.

g Picture arrangement: logically rearranging a disordered set of pictures.

h Object assembly: completing three jigsaw puzzles as fast as possible.

i Digit symbol substitution: coding random digits at speed according to a given key.

j Block design: translating a small, two-dimensional design into a full-scale design, using colored cubes.

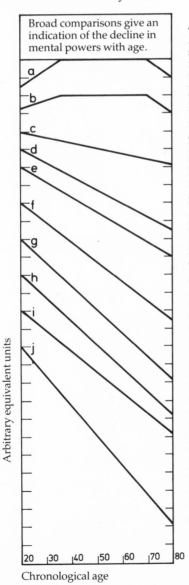

Broad comparisons give an indication of the decline in mental powers with age.

Arbitrary equivalent units

20 30 40 50 60 70 80

Chronological age

4 Decline of the Senses

Ability to hear high-pitched sounds declines with age as nerves die off at the basal turn of the inner ear. In their 20s most people can no longer hear bats' high-pitched squeaks (**a**). By their 50s, they miss the highest tones of songbirds (**b**). In old age some people cannot even hear the treble notes of a piano (**c**), though increased volume helps to make these sounds more audible. More annoyingly, speech may become difficult to understand. Here, though, reduced intelligence and other factors play a part. More men than women suffer loss of hearing. The left ear is often more affected than the right.

As aging knocks out sensory receptors, those detecting smell and taste suffer heavy casualties. The diagram shows the numbers of taste buds left in the trench wall of a single papilla at the ages of 20 (**d**), 60 (**e**), and 80 (**f**). By 80, sensitivity to salt and sugar has been much diminished. Meanwhile, olfactory receptors have been dying off since birth (**g**). By 20 (**h**), 18 per cent are already lost. From 20 to 60 (**i**), 44 per cent disappear. By their early 80s (**j**) people retain little more than one fourth of the olfactory receptors that they were born with, so their sense of smell is much diminished.

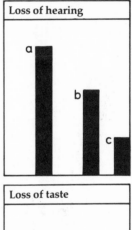

Loss of hearing

Loss of taste

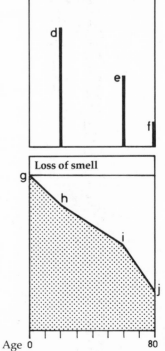

Loss of smell

Age 0   80

© DIAGRAM

Chapter 4

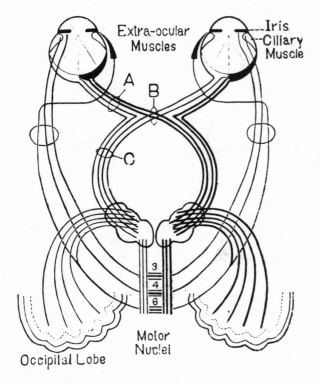

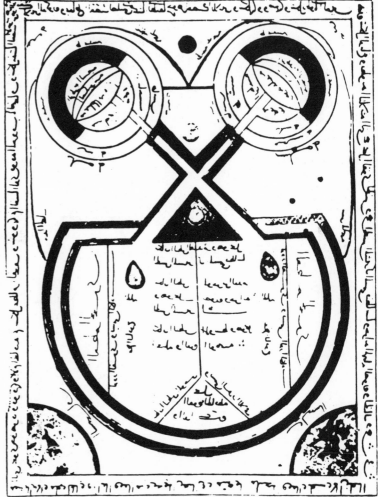

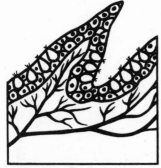

НИТЕВИДНЫЙ

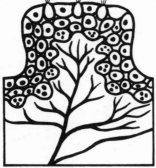

ГРИБОВИДНЫЙ

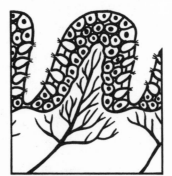

ЛИСТОВИДНЫЙ

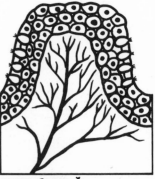

ВАЛИКОВИДНЫЙ

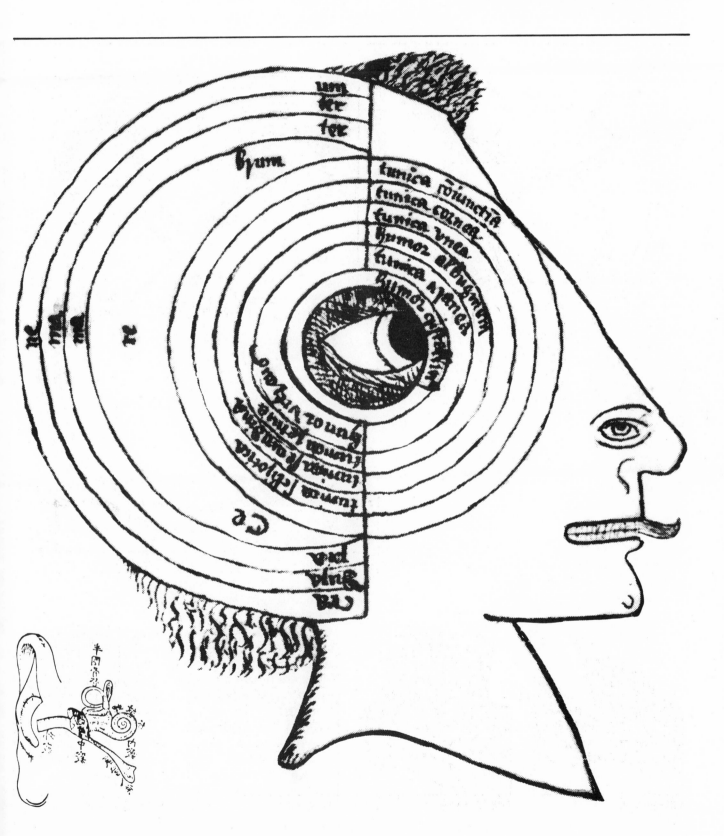

Touch, Pain, and Temperature

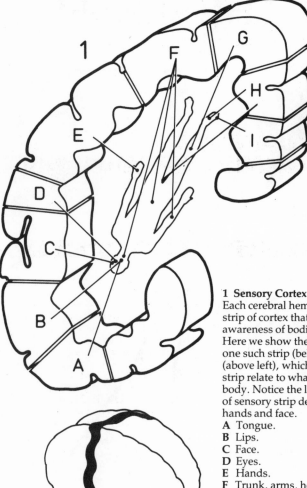

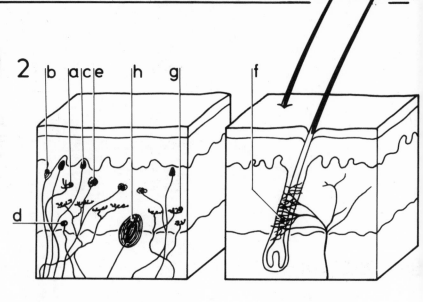

1 Sensory Cortex
Each cerebral hemisphere has a strip of cortex that handles awareness of bodily sensations. Here we show the location of one such strip (below left) and, (above left), which parts of that strip relate to what parts of the body. Notice the large regions of sensory strip dealing with hands and face.
A Tongue.
B Lips.
C Face.
D Eyes.
E Hands.
F Trunk, arms, head.
G Legs.
H Feet, genitals.
I Toes.

2 Skin Receptors
In this diagram, numbered items represent types of nerve ending found at different levels in the skin. Each type of ending is sensitive to one kind of stimulus or to a group of stimuli. The free nerve endings and beaded nerve net probably detect pain. Merkel's disks, Meissner's corpuscles and hair organs sense touch. (The first two are commonest in hairless areas of skin.) Krause's end bulbs specialize in sensing cold, while Ruffini corpuscles detect heat. The rather deep-seated Pacinian corpuscles are pressure receptors, also sensitive to stretching and vibration.

a Free nerve endings.
b Merkel's disks.
c Meissner's corpuscles.
d Beaded nerve net.
e Krause's end bulbs.
f Hair organs.
g Ruffini corpuscles.
h Pacinian corpuscles.

People traditionally speak of the five senses: sight, hearing, smell, taste and feeling. In fact, the body contains nerve endings sensitive to light, sound, touch, pressure, heat, cold, hunger, thirst, pain, fatigue and other stimuli. The information that they feed into the spinal cord and brain enables us to monitor the world around us, and, to a large extent, to know what is going on inside our bodies. Often unaware that we are doing so, we respond to the information brought in by our senses in ways that help to keep us alive – for example by stepping from the path of an oncoming truck or drinking when we feel thirsty.

Scientists identify three main types of nerve ending designed to gather information: exteroceptors handling information fed in from outside the body; interoceptors, reporting changes deep inside the body; and proprioceptors, that tell us about joint and muscle movements.

Strongly stimulated receptors inhibit those around them and send signals to spinal cord or brainstem. The signals may travel to the thalamus which sorts and forwards information to the higher centers of the brain. But unimportant signals are ignored, and may be discontinued.

There are hundreds of thousands of sensitive exteroceptor units on the body's surface. Most are concentrated in certain places – especially the lips, tongue tip and finger pads. The large brain area designed to handle sensations from the face, hands and feet shows the importance of these parts of the body for probing and sensing the outside world.

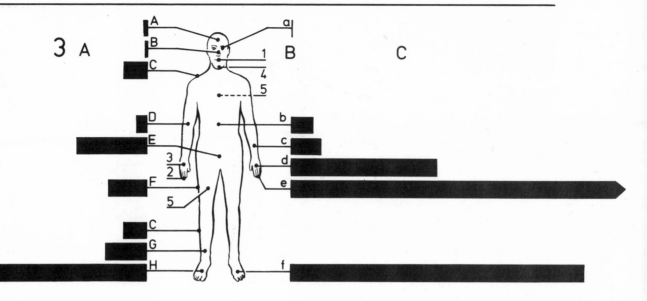

3A Touch Sensitivity

Different areas of skin vary in sensitivity to the effects of pressure. This diagram shows relative pressures needed to evoke a sensation of touch in eight prodded areas. The longer a bar, the greater the pressure. Pressures range from 2–250g per mm² (2.8–356lb per in²).

A	Forehead	3g/mm²
B	Nose	2g/mm²
C	Shoulder, calf	16g/mm²
D	Arm	7g/mm²
E	Loins	48g/mm²
F	Outer thigh	26g/mm²
G	Shin	28g/mm²
H	Thick sole	250g/mm²

3B Touch Discrimination

Blindfold, most people can locate a single pinprick. But two pricks are felt as one unless far enough apart. The minimum distance for two-point discrimination varies partly with the local density of touch receptors. The right-hand diagram shows actual minimum distances for two-point discrimination on parts of the body numbered as above.

1	Tongue tip	1mm
2	Fingertip	2mm
3	Back of hand	32mm
4	Back of neck	54mm
5	Middle of back and front of thigh	67mm

3C Sensing Pain

Pricking any area of skin may reveal 10 times more "pain spots" than centers sensitive to touch. But here, too, some parts of the body surface are more sensitive than others. Fingertips need three times the pressure that evokes pain in the back of the hand. Our diagram includes relative pressures needed to evoke a sense of pain in six areas. Pressures illustrated go from 0.2–300g per mm² (0.28–427lb per in²).

a	Cornea	0.2g/mm²
b	Abdomen	15 g/mm²
c	Front of forearm	20g/mm²
d	Back of hand	100g/mm²
e	Fingertip	300g/mm²
f	Sole	200g/mm²

Skin contains two main types of receptor: mechanoreceptors and thermoreceptors. Mechanoreceptors sense touch or pressure, firing off nerve impulses when touch or pressure tends to push them out of shape. Most touch receptors take the form of bulbs or corpuscles. Others are nerve endings forming webs around the roots of hairs. Touching a hair moves it like a tiny lever. This magnifies the "touch" effect and activates the so-called hair organs.

Some free nerve endings – those formed like tiny branching twigs – may be sensitive to touch, pressure and pain. But intense pressure on other kinds of nerve ending may trigger pain as well. Pain seems related to the size of nerve affected. A mild electric stimulus to large nerve fibers below the skin gives a harmless rubbing sensation. A stronger stimulus affects narrower nerves, producing a sensation of impending pain. An even stronger stimulus affects still smaller fibers and real pain is felt. Stimulating the smallest nerve fibers causes excruciating pain.

One kind of mechanoreceptor may produce several sensations, according to the stimuli it registers. Lightly agitated touch receptors produce a tickling sensation. Mildly stimulated pain receptors make us itch. We sense vibration through receptors that also deal with pressure. Thermoreceptors – nerve endings sensitive to heat and cold – come in two main kinds, called Krause's end bulbs and Ruffini corpuscles. The first type registers cold, the second, heat.

©DIAGRAM

Our Inner Senses

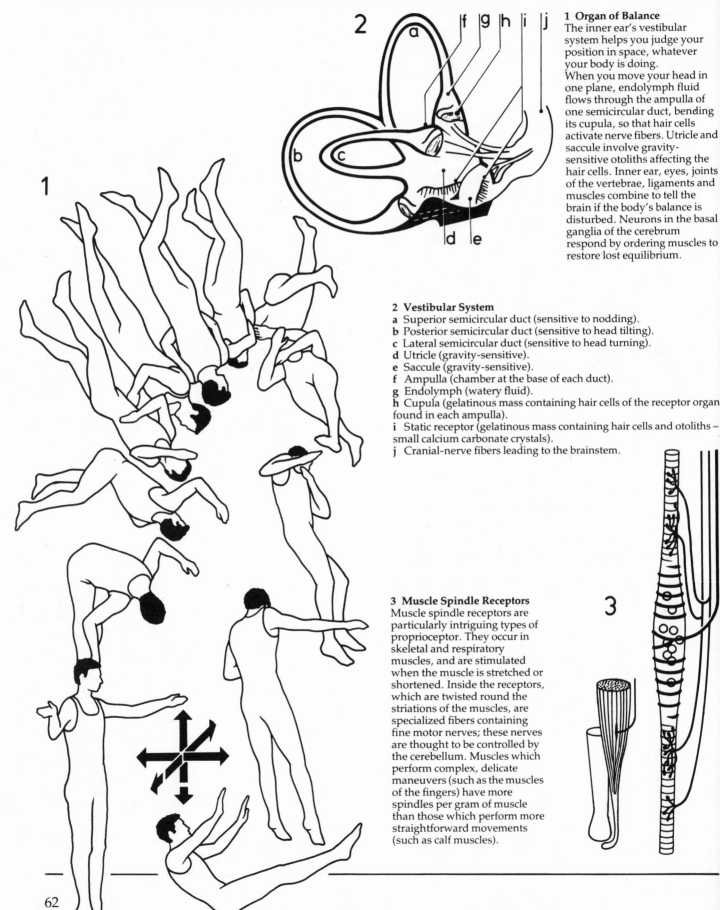

1 Organ of Balance
The inner ear's vestibular system helps you judge your position in space, whatever your body is doing.

When you move your head in one plane, endolymph fluid flows through the ampulla of one semicircular duct, bending its cupula, so that hair cells activate nerve fibers. Utricle and saccule involve gravity-sensitive otoliths affecting the hair cells. Inner ear, eyes, joints of the vertebrae, ligaments and muscles combine to tell the brain if the body's balance is disturbed. Neurons in the basal ganglia of the cerebrum respond by ordering muscles to restore lost equilibrium.

2 Vestibular System
a Superior semicircular duct (sensitive to nodding).
b Posterior semicircular duct (sensitive to head tilting).
c Lateral semicircular duct (sensitive to head turning).
d Utricle (gravity-sensitive).
e Saccule (gravity-sensitive).
f Ampulla (chamber at the base of each duct).
g Endolymph (watery fluid).
h Cupula (gelatinous mass containing hair cells of the receptor organ found in each ampulla).
i Static receptor (gelatinous mass containing hair cells and otoliths – small calcium carbonate crystals).
j Cranial-nerve fibers leading to the brainstem.

3 Muscle Spindle Receptors
Muscle spindle receptors are particularly intriguing types of proprioceptor. They occur in skeletal and respiratory muscles, and are stimulated when the muscle is stretched or shortened. Inside the receptors, which are twisted round the striations of the muscles, are specialized fibers containing fine motor nerves; these nerves are thought to be controlled by the cerebellum. Muscles which perform complex, delicate maneuvers (such as the muscles of the fingers) have more spindles per gram of muscle than those which perform more straightforward movements (such as calf muscles).

Nerve endings sensitive to movement or pressure and buried deep inside the body feed the spinal cord and brain information vital for working of the muscles that automatically adjust the position of the body and its limbs, and control the function of internal organs.

The vestibular system of the inner ear helps us keep our balance, even with our eyes shut. Its looped semicircular ducts are three tubes at right angles, communicating with the saclike saccule and utricle. Each structure has hair cells linked to nerve fibers. Head movements set fluid flowing through the ducts and sacs, moving hair cells that trigger signals from nerve fibers to the brain via the eighth cranial nerve. Different movements of the head activate different sets of fibers.

Between them, the semicircular ducts register nodding, tilting and turning of the head. The saccule and utricle tell the brain the attitude of the head in relation to the pull of gravity. This is largely why we can stand or walk in the dark.

Picking up a cup or taking a step is a simple-seeming operation. Yet its success depends on batteries of signals fired from proprioceptors, informing spinal cord and brain which muscles are relaxed and which contracted, and sending data about the changing angle formed by bones at each joint as you bend or stretch a leg or an arm.

Three kinds of proprioceptor are involved. Joint receptors in the capsule surrounding each joint register how much and how fast it moves. Golgi tendon receptors on ligaments joining muscles to bones signal muscular contraction or passive stretch. Muscle spindle receptors in each muscle tell these apart and measure the amount of a contraction. Between them, then, three types of proprioceptor help to maintain limb positions or smoothly alter them – as local reflex actions or as movements consciously directed by the brain. Deep inside the body a whole orchestra of specialized receptors, largely coordinated by the lower centers of the brain, operates to ensure the body's vital functions go on working.

Thus muscle spindle receptors help to control the shortening of respiratory muscles that work to keep the lungs in action.

Pressure receptors, alias baroreceptors, in the walls of the heart and large blood vessels respond to stretching and so warn the central nervous system of changes in blood pressure. If this rises, the receptors fire off signals faster. The brain then slows the heart rate and lets blood vessels dilate so blood can flow more easily. If blood pressure falls, the receptors send fewer signals. The brain then constricts smaller arteries and makes the heart beat more powerfully.

Osmoreceptors in the hypothalamus and lower brainstem sense changes in the osmotic pressure produced by salts and proteins in the blood. The hypothalamus responds by issuing instructions to the kidneys to adjust osmotic pressure by varying the amount of fluid in the body. Also in the hypothalamus are thermoreceptor cells sensitive to blood temperature changes of less than 0.1°C.

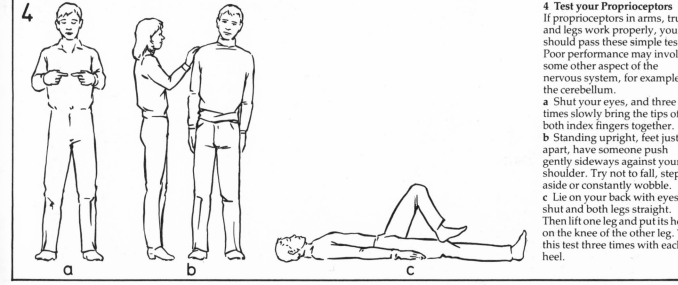

4 Test your Proprioceptors
If proprioceptors in arms, trunk and legs work properly, you should pass these simple tests. Poor performance may involve some other aspect of the nervous system, for example the cerebellum.
a Shut your eyes, and three times slowly bring the tips of both index fingers together.
b Standing upright, feet just apart, have someone push gently sideways against your shoulder. Try not to fall, step aside or constantly wobble.
c Lie on your back with eyes shut and both legs straight. Then lift one leg and put its heel on the knee of the other leg. Try this test three times with each heel.

Sight

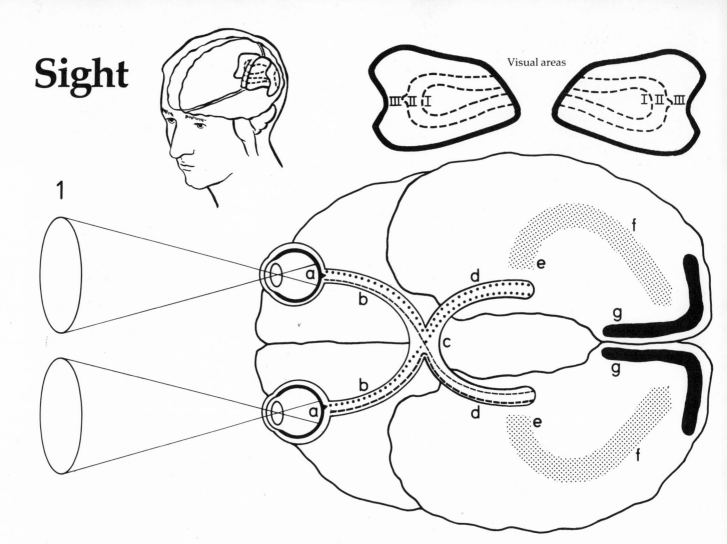

Visual areas

1 Eyes and Brain
This view of the underside of the brain shows the visual pathways from eyes to occipital cortex at the back of the brain (shown in three dimensions on the inset diagram above).

Eye Control
Cranial nerves control eyeball movements. Both eyes can work together to focus on and follow one object. (The back of the brain fuses both views of the object to give an illusion of depth.)

Optic Chiasma
At this cross-over point, optic fibers from the inner half of each retina cross to the opposite half of the brain. Fibers from the retinas' outer halves do not cross.
a Retina.
b Optic nerve.
c Optic chiasma.
d Optic tract.

Visual Cortex
From the two geniculate bodies, optic radiation fibers fan out and finish up at the visual part of the occipital cortex. Here we "see" – ie register electrochemical impulses that arrive from the eyes.
e Geniculate body.
f Optic radiation.
g Visual cortex.

Sight involves mechanisms that convert light waves arriving from objects into electrochemical impulses that reach special regions at the back of the cerebral cortex. No other sense involves so many nerve cells, which shows just how much we need sight to learn about our surroundings.
Vision starts with the eyes – two jelly-filled balls set in the front of the skull, rotated by sets of muscles, and linked by thick optic nerves with the back of the cerebral hemispheres.
Incoming light rays pass right through the eye. The rays are bent by the lens as they enter the eye via the cornea and travel on through the aqueous humor. After entering the pupil (an adjustable hole) they are bent and inverted by the lens, finally arriving at the retina ("net").

This thin web of nerve cells at the back of the eyeball is a mobile, specialized offshoot of the brain. It is made back to front, for light has to penetrate outer layers of retinal nerve cells before reaching the photoreceptor ("light-sensing") cells at the back of the retina. There are two types of photoreceptor: 6 million relatively short, thick, color-sensitive cones; and 125 million longer, thinner rods, which allow us to see in dim light, but just in shades of gray.
Light falling on rods and cones affects light-sensitive pigments, triggering chemical changes that send coded signals from the rods and cones through the optic nerves deep inside the brain. Nerve fibers are so organized that each bit of the image formed on the retina travels in code through

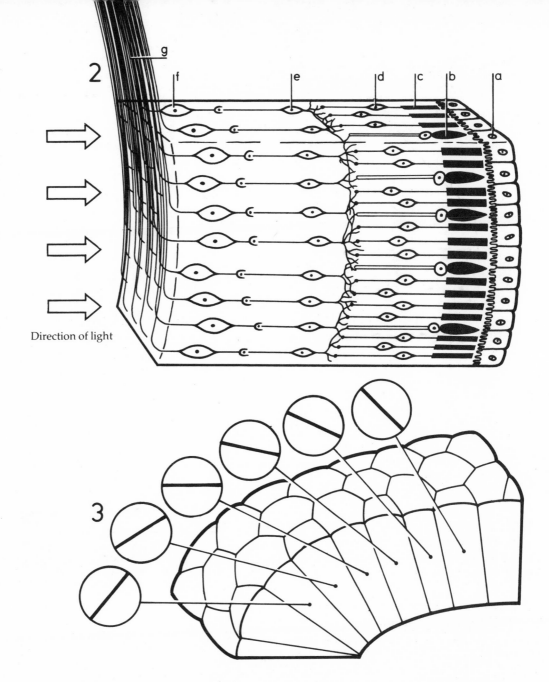

2 How a Retina Works

This diagram depicts a much enlarged section of a retina – a cup-shaped brain "bud," designed back to front. Light must pass through layers of nerve cells before reaching the rods and cones. There, light triggers electrochemical impulses that go back through the layers of nerve cells that lead to the optic nerve. The pigment cells prevent spread of bright light between the rod and cone cells.

a Pigment cells.
b Cones.
c Rods.
d Rod nucleus.
e Intermediate neuron.
f Integrating neuron.
g Optic nerve.

Direction of light

3 Inside the Visual Cortex

Mapping visual cortex cells (right) shows that each cell column only reacts to a specific visual stimulus (shown circled). In this example, different columns react to lines at different angles. Researchers divide visual cortex cells into three main types. "Simple" cells in visual area I flanking the brain's central fissure register bright lines or dark bars at specific angles. "Complex" and "hypercomplex" cells occupy nearby visual areas II and III. Complex cells detect edges and movement in certain directions. Hypercomplex cells detect corners.

the inside of the skull in an orderly fashion. Somehow, the whole image is reassembled (still coded of course) after reaching the cortex of the brain's occipital lobe.

The journey to the back of the brain is astonishingly complex. Near the back of the eyes, both optic nerves meet at the so-called optic chiasma ("crossing"). Here, nerve fibers from the part of each retina nearest the nose cross over. Thus the resulting left optic tract carries data about objects from the right-hand side of the field of vision, and the right optic tract takes signals from objects seen on the left.

Continuing back through the cerebral hemispheres, each optic tract reaches a lateral geniculate body ("bent like a knee") – a relay station in a thalamus. From there optic signals pass on through the optic radiation – a ribbon of nerve fibers ending at the primary visual cortex, the back inside edge of each cerebral hemisphere.

Research shows that here, in the primary visual cortex (visual area I), different columns of brain cells register signals from different parts of the retina. Signals received here pass on to nearby visual areas II and III for further refinement. In each visual area, special cells react only to signals produced by special visual stimuli – for instance lines at particular angles, or movements in certain directions.

Between them, these visual areas process visual signals in ways that help us to grasp the sizes, shapes and positions of the objects that we see.

© DIAGRAM

Hearing

The function of our ears is largely to convert sounds produced by pressure waves in air into electrochemical signals that travel to the brain's temporal lobes – the "hearing centers" where sound signals are interpreted and understood. Each ear has three main parts: the inner, middle and outer ear. The outer ear, or pinna, includes a fleshy, cuplike auricle, collecting sound waves and funneling them into the external auditory canal – a hole in the side of the head. Sound waves travel about 1½ inches (3.8cm) through this tunnel to a six-sided "box" – the middle ear.

In the middle ear, sound waves vibrate the eardrum – a frail sheet of tissue guarding the middle ear's entrance. The eardrum in turn vibrates a sequence of tiny, movable bones: the malleus ("hammer"), incus ("anvil") and stapes ("stirrup"), the smallest bone in the body. Sound vibrations also reach the inner ear through the bones of the skull, though less effectively.

The vibrating stapes plunges in and out of the oval window that leads to the inner ear – a complex system of fluid-filled membranous chambers including the cochlea, a structure coiled like a snail's shell and divided in two lengthwise by the so-called basilar membrane. The stapes sends waves through fluid in the cochlea. These waves make the basilar membrane vibrate. In turn this agitates the organ of Corti – a tunnel bounded by rods flanked by thousands of sensitive hairs attached to 30,000 nerve fibers.

When the hairs vibrate the nerve fibers send signals (corresponding to the pitch and volume of the sound heard by the outer ear) through the eighth cranial (acoustic) nerve to the brainstem. There, many of the nerve fibers from each side of the head cross over before taking signals up through the cerebral hemispheres to the tops of the brain's temporal lobes for analysis. Signals from each ear thus reach both temporal lobes. This means that if one lobe suffers damage its owner need not become deaf in one ear.

Signals arriving at the brain from both ears help us to pinpoint where the sounds have come from. The lowest sounds man can hear are produced by sound waves with a frequency of 20 cycles per second. Waves of 20,000 cycles per second produce the highest audible sounds. The faintest sounds we hear are rated at 1 decibel – a unit of intensity based on sound-wave amplitude. Noise above 100 decibels can damage the inner ear. Intense sound, aging, head injury and some diseases can all cause sensorineural, ie perceptive, deafness.

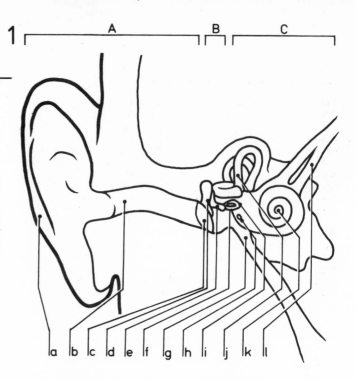

1 Parts of the Ear
Ear structures form three groups, as shown (above).
A The outer ear includes the pinna and the external auditory canal.
B The middle ear includes the eardrum, malleus, incus, stapes, and eustachian tube (adjusting air pressure in the middle ear).
C The inner ear features the round window, oval window, organ of balance and cochlea linked to the auditory nerve.

a Pinna.
b External auditory canal.
c Eardrum.
d Malleus.
e Incus.
f Stapes.
g Eustachian tube.
h Round window.
i Oval window.
j Organ of balance.
k Cochlea.
l Acoustic nerve.

The diagram (below) shows in simplified fashion routes by which signals flow from ears to brainstem, then up to the temporal lobes of the cerebral hemispheres, where the brain consciously registers sounds.

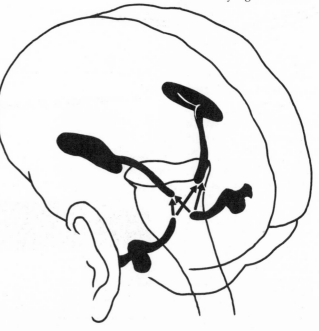

2 Shown here is an enlarged cross-section of structures inside the cochlea.
a Vestibular canal.
b Vestibular membrane.
c Cochlear duct.
d Basilar membrane.
e Organ of Corti.
f Acoustic nerve.
g Tympanic canal.

3 The key cochlear structures are here shown magnified.
h Hair cells.
i Rods of Corti.
j Tectorial membrane.
k Basilar membrane.

Inside the Cochlea

In the cochlea pressure waves arriving from the middle ear trigger electrochemical impulses to be passed to the brain. Cross-section 2 shows cochlear structures involved. Pressure waves in perilymph fluid inside the vestibular canal vibrate the vestibular membrane, which displaces the fluid-filled cochlear duct. In turn this displaces the basilar membrane and the attached organ of Corti. Section 3 shows this last part in detail. Rods of Corti support hair cells whose ends reach up to the tectorial membrane. Vibrating hair cells send signals through nerve fibers to the brain.

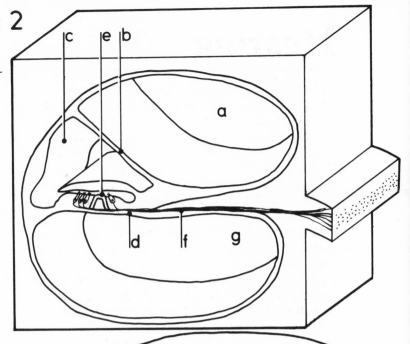

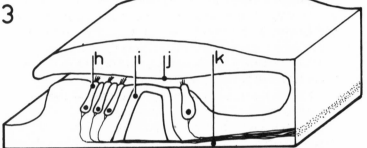

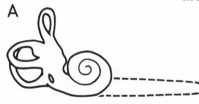

4 Basilar Membrane

A cochlea (**A**) is also shown from the inside, straightened and magnified (**B**). Pressure waves of differing frequency vibrate different sections of its basilar membrane (**C**). High-frequency waves die out near the membrane's narrow base. Low-frequency waves reach maximum amplitude at the broad far end. Hair cells linked to the auditory nerve react only over that part of the membrane where waves "peak." This is how the brain can tell if a sound is high pitched or low.
a Pressure waves.
b Basilar membrane.
c Basilar membrane.
d High-frequency waves.
e Low-frequency waves.

Base

1,500–20,000 cps

500–1,500 cps

20–500 cps

Tip

First turn

Second turn

Third turn

© DIAGRAM

Smell and Taste

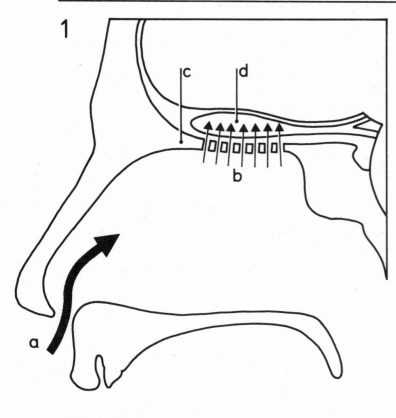

Sense organs called chemoreceptors enable us to tell salt from sugar, a fragrance from a stench. Chemoreceptors identify substances just by touching some of the molecules that they are made of – but only if the substances have been dissolved. This is why olfactory receptors and taste buds are always kept moist.

Our millions of smell receptors lie concentrated in two olfactory membranes – one in each nasal cavity behind the bridge of the nose. The two take up only about 1 square inch (6.5sq cm) but contain 10–20 million olfactory nerve endings. Each of these ends in 20 threadlike filaments. The total area of filaments may exceed that of your skin. Only 2 per cent of the air you breathe in passes over these receptors. Yet they are so sensitive that a human nose can detect 32 millionths of 1000 millionths of 1 ounce (28.4g) of musk.

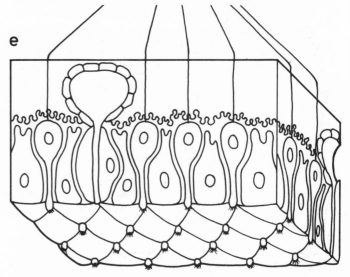

1 Olfactory Bulb
Scent particles entering the nose with breathed-in air stimulate smell receptors at the top of the nasal cavity. From there, the receptors send electrochemical signals through perforations in the ethmoid bone's cribriform plate to an olfactory bulb linked to the rest of the brain's limbic system.

a Air entering nose.
b Electrochemical signals from smell receptors.
c Cribriform plate.
d Olfactory bulb.
e Smell receptors shown greatly enlarged. Each olfactory nerve ending has 20 threadlike filaments in touch with the nasal cavity.

2 Stereochemical Theory
This theory of olfaction suggests that different scent receptor sites act like locks entered only by special keys: appropriately shaped scent molecules. The diagram (below) shows supposed shapes of receptor sites that accept five "primary" odors.

a Minty.
b Ethereal.
c Floral.
d Musky.
e Camphoraceous.

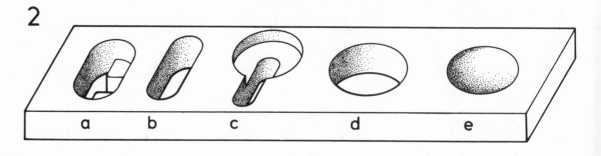

All smells are evidently based on only seven primary odors. Theory has it that their molecules have different shapes fitting hollows in the smell receptors, as different keys fit different locks. Someone with a keen sense of smell can identify as many as 10,000 odors, most probably produced by combinations of the supposed seven primaries. Somehow, scent molecules reaching chemoreceptor filaments trigger nerve signals given off by cells growing down inside the olfactory membrane. Nerve fibers carrying these signals join inside the skull to form two olfactory bulbs that lead directly to the brain's limbic system.

Our sense of taste is far less acute than our sense of smell. Evidently we need 25,000 times more of a chemical compound to taste it than we do to smell it. This is partly because our taste chemoreceptors are far less sensitive than the olfactory receptors in the nose.

Taste buds occur mostly on the tongue, but also on palate, throat and tonsils. An adult may have 9000 taste buds, a baby many more. Each taste bud comprises groups of taste-sensitive cells. Each cell has tiny taste-sensitive hairs and links with several nerves sending signals to the brainstem. As many as 200 taste buds grow on each of the scores of papillae ("pimples") that make the top of the tongue feel rough.

The tongue registers only four main tastes: salt, sweet, sour and bitter; but combinations of these (plus pain, touch and temperature sensations) produce the variety of flavors we experience. Diverse tastes and temperatures register most strongly on different areas of the tongue, and travel to the brainstem via different nerves. From there they go to the thalamus and then the cortex.

3

3 Taste Receptors
Taste receptors called taste buds are scattered over much of the tongue. The diagram (right) shows taste buds, two much enlarged, lining the walls of a saliva-filled trench between two papillae (tiny lumps that cover the surface of the tongue). Each taste bud contains taste-sensitive cells ending in hairs that send signals back to the brain. Certain parts of the tongue (left) are especially sensitive to one or other of four basic tastes:
a Bitter.
b Sour.
c Salty.
d Sweet.

4 Pathways to the Brain
From taste buds in the tongue, "taste" signals speed through gustatory nerves to centers in the lower brainstem. From there signals go to the thalamus, then on to the cerebral cortex. Because olfactory nerve fibers cross over in the medulla, taste signals from each side of the tongue are interpreted in the opposite brain hemisphere.
a Tongue.
b Medulla.
c Thalamus.
d Cortex.

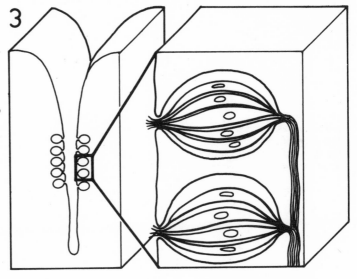

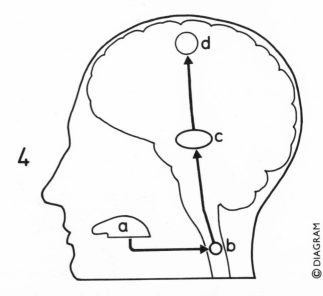

© DIAGRAM

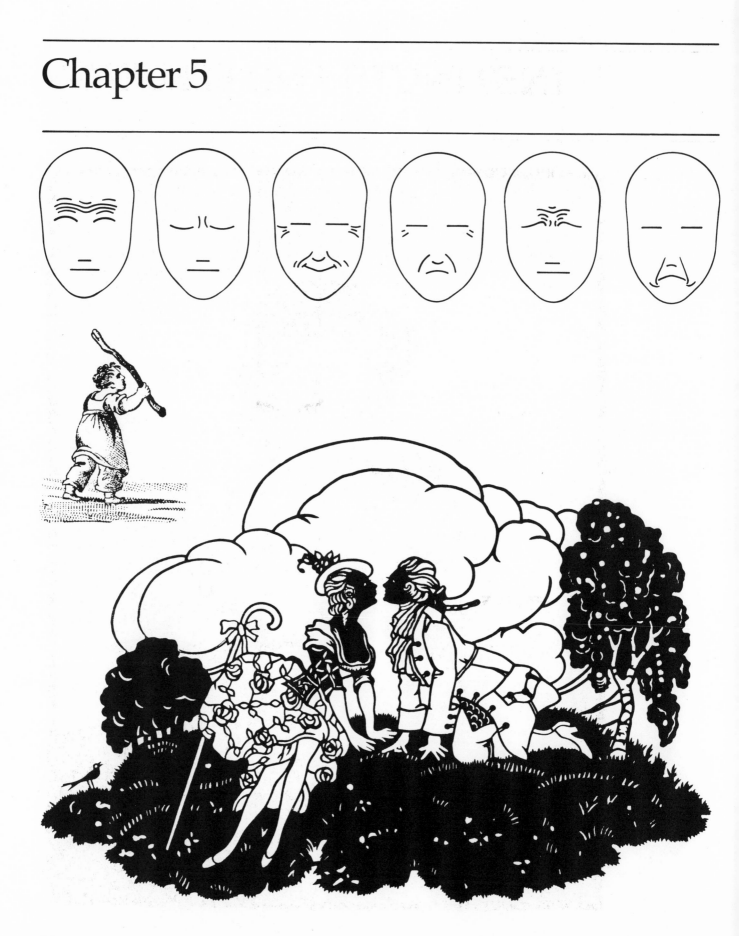

Chapter 5

INSTINCTS AND FEELINGS

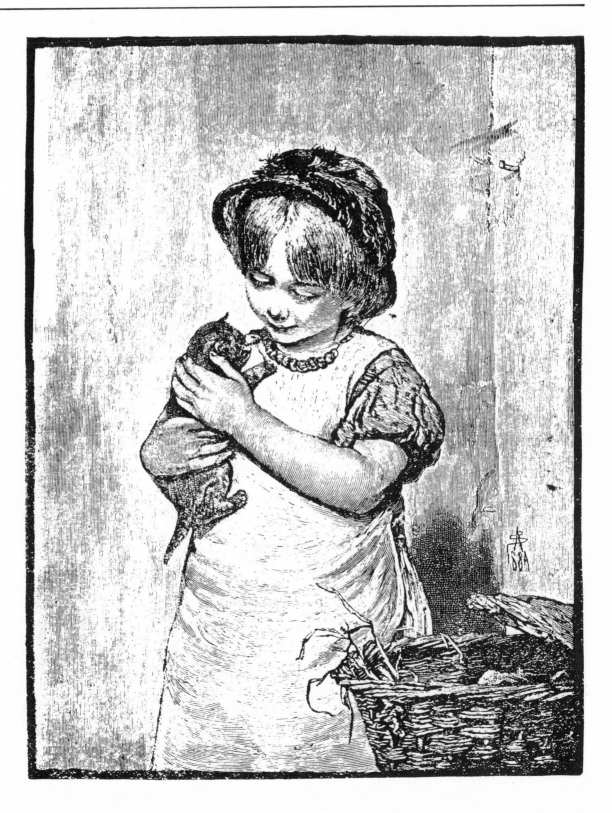

Reflexes

Unlike animals with very simple brains, we partially control the workings of our bodies. Yet many activities depend on built-in circuits of the nervous system that operate automatically, without reference to the higher centers of the brain. This can have two advantages. First, it speeds up muscle movements in emergency. Second, because this automatic movement involves few nerve cells it frees others for coping with more complicated problems.

Sneezing, coughing, jerking the hand away from a hot radiator are three such reflex actions.

The simplest type of reflex involves a chain of just two neurons. For instance, if a doctor's hammer taps the tendon below your kneecap, a sensory neuron informs a motor neuron in the spinal cord. The motor neuron responds by making a muscle contract to jerk the knee up suddenly. Other simple jerk reflexes involve the ankle, foot and elbow.

Most kinds of reflex are more complicated than the knee jerk. This is partly due to interneuron "go-betweens" in the spinal cord, bridging gaps between sensory and motor neurons. An interneuron may connect with many more neurons. Such multiple connections can trigger reflexes involving groups of muscles. But while neurons tell some muscles to contract, other muscles receive "don't act" instructions. This helps to stop opposing muscles canceling each other out.

Not all reflexes are independent of the brain.

Logically enough, the brain itself handles those involving organs in the head. The brainstem manages reflexes that control the size of the pupils of the eyes, turn the head toward a sound, keep the eyes smoothly fixed on an object while the head nods or turns, and help adjust the falling body's attitude in relation to gravity.

The brainstem is involved in some reflexes far below the head – helping to contract muscles in abdomen, inner thigh and foot when certain parts of these are stroked or scratched.

Similarly, belching, coughing, yawning, sneezing, vomiting are reflex actions built into the lowest levels of the brain. Surprisingly, all of these reflexes work well in anencephalic babies born with a bag of fluid where the cerebrum should be.

The brain's hypothalamus is crucial to some so-called hormonal reflexes, for example the flow of milk in nursing mothers. Other hormonal reflexes, such as those involving gastrointestinal hormones, do not involve the central nervous system.

Many reflexes protect the body from, or adjust it to, its surroundings. Some do both. If you step on a tack with a bare foot, contracting flexor muscles bend your knee to pull the foot away. But reflex bending of one knee triggers reflex straightening of the other, which helps you keep your balance. All this occurs before the thalamus inside your brain has even noticed pain.

Meanwhile, autonomic reflexes are always acting to control breathing, blood supply and so on, to maintain the status quo inside the body.

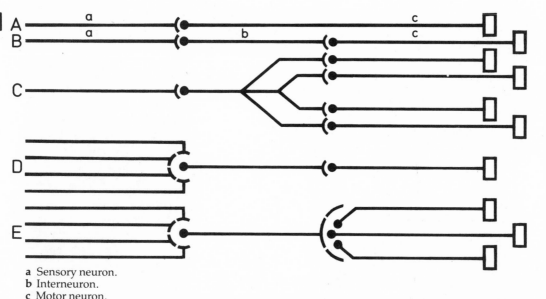

1 A

a Sensory neuron.
b Interneuron.
c Motor neuron.

1 Types of Reflex
Some reflexes are very simple, but usually they are quite complicated, and involve sending detailed sets of instructions to other areas of the body.
A The most elementary reflex: a sensory neuron (**a**) sends a message to a motor neuron (**c**) at the same level in the spinal cord.
B More often, sensory and motor neurons are linked by a second neuron (**b**).
C An interneuron connects one sensory neuron with several motor neurons.
D Several sensory neurons are linked by interneuron with one motor neuron.
E Information from several sensory neurons is relayed to levels higher and lower in the spinal cord.

Reflex Routes

Reflexes are the most basic functions of the central nervous system. Vital muscle movements, such as those involved in breathing, are all controlled by reflexes, and though we may be aware of some of the actions these nerve loops perform for us, others occur without our knowledge.

2 The knee jerk is a very simple reflex which is carried out by just two neurons (near right). A sensory neuron (**a**) carries a message to the spinal cord, saying that it has picked up a stretch of the tendon below the knee. This is relayed directly to a motor neuron (**b**) which contracts the muscle, swinging the leg.

3 Most reflexes are more complex than the knee jerk and involve interneurons (**b**) within the spinal cord. In this case, pain registered by a sensory nerve in the skin (**a**) when it senses heat triggers a quick reaction from a motor nerve (**c**) in the arm, which draws the hand away. Pain messages (**d**) are sent up to the brain, but the reflex has acted before the brain has even registered this impression.

4 If you happen to step on a tack with your bare foot, a widespread reflex response takes place. A sensory neuron (**a**), registering the pain in your foot, links up at the spinal cord with a network of interneurons (**b**) which send messages to several muscles through motor neurons (**c**). The result is that one muscle bends your knee to pull the foot away while, at the same time, other leg muscles act to help you keep your balance. Messages passing up the spinal cord produce movements of head and arms, together with the involuntary "ouch!"

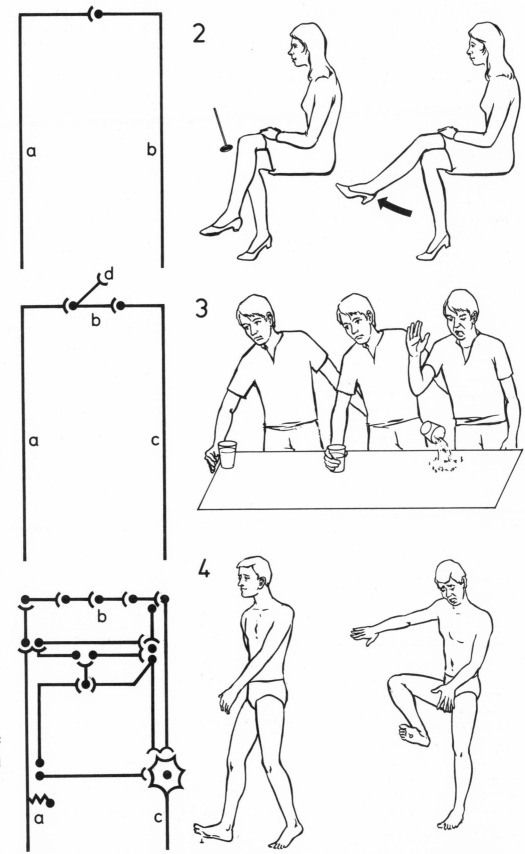

©DIAGRAM

Regulating Body Functions

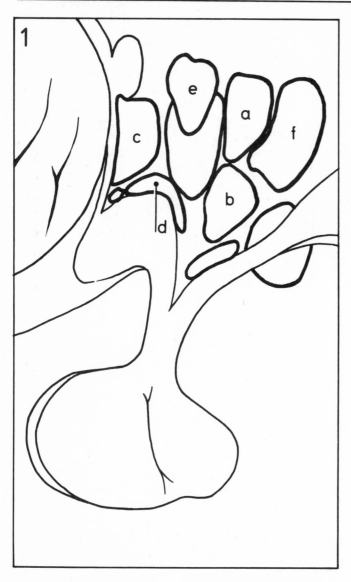

To stay alive we need controlled conditions in our bodies. We die if the body core becomes too hot or cold, or if body tissues get too dry, or waterlogged, or starved of food or oxygen. Special regions of the brain prevent all this by regulating body functions to maintain homeostasis – internal equilibrium. These brain-directed checks and balances work automatically, and we are usually unaware of most of them.

Muscular activities like breathing and heartbeat depend on groups of nerve cells in the lower brainstem. For instance, so-called inspiratory centers control breathing in, while expiratory centers handle breathing out.

However, the body's chief controller is the hypothalamus, bridging nervous and endocrine (hormonal) systems, and a kingpin of mechanisms based on feedback principles. Much of its work consists of responding to chemical imbalance in blood by telling the pituitary gland to issue hormones that correct these errors.

Special regions of the hypothalamus control different bodily activities. If heat-sensitive nerve cells in the preoptic nucleus near the front of the hypothalamus receive "too cold" signals from heat sensors in the skin, the hypothalamus tells the pituitary gland to yield a chemical that triggers the release of thyroid hormone in the blood. Thyroid hormone in turn steps up the body's heat production. Meanwhile, blood vessels in the skin contract, reducing loss of body heat by radiation. "Too hot" signals reaching the hypothalamus can make the skin sweat and its blood vessels dilate, so

1 The Hypothalamus
Lying at the base of the brain, the hypothalamus (above) acts as the body's special control center, monitoring vital functions like regulation of body temperature and appetite. Changes in the chemical balance of the blood are responded to by the hypothalamus which then instructs the pituitary gland to release appropriate hormonal messengers to remedy the situation. Certain areas of the hypothalamus, keyed on the diagram above, are responsible for monitoring specific bodily functions:

a The dorsomedial nucleus controls aggression.
b The ventromedial nucleus is an appestat – that is, it controls food intake.
c The preoptic nucleus at the front of the gland serves as a thermostat.
d The supraoptic nucleus is associated with thirst.
e The paraventricular nucleus also monitors water in the body, and stimulates production of a hormone that makes the womb contract after childbirth.
f The posterior nucleus controls the sex drive.

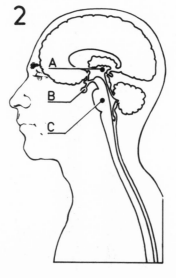

2 Body Regulators
The diagram (left) shows the relative positions of the hypothalamus (**A**), pituitary (**B**) and brainstem (**C**). Correct functioning of all these areas is vital to maintain homeostasis – internal equilibrium. The hypothalamus and pituitary work in tandem, with hypothalamus acting as a body sensor and pituitary yielding chemicals to rectify any imbalance. The brainstem controls important functions like respiration – breathing in and out.

helping the body to lose heat by evaporation and radiation.

While the front of the hypothalamus serves as a thermostat, regions at the sides are appestats, controlling food intake. Stimulating so-called hunger sites with electrodes provokes overeating in fully fed laboratory animals; stimulating nearby satiety sites robs even ravenous animals of appetite. Between them, our own satiety and hunger sites normally prevent us starving or overeating. How hungry we feel at any time depends largely on the amount of glucose circulating in the blood as monitored within the brain.

Controlling the body's water content is another vital task accomplished by the hypothalamus. If the body's water content falls, salt concentration builds up in the blood, and special sensors warn the supraoptic region of the hypothalamus. One consequence is feeling thirsty. Another is release of large amounts of vasopressin or antidiuretic hormone (ADH) from the pituitary gland into the bloodstream. This makes kidneys reabsorb water otherwise scheduled for evacuation as urine. Reabsorption in turn helps reduce the further loss of water from the body.

When too much water accumulates inside the body the hypothalamus registers a reduced salt level in the blood, the pituitary yields less ADH, and more water flows from kidneys to bladder.

In one way or another the hypothalamus regulates most processes essential to life.

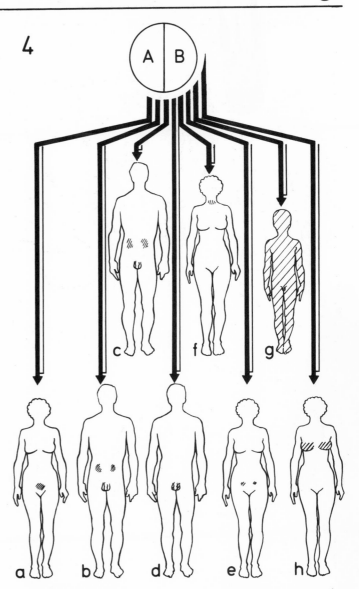

3 How the Hypothalamus Acts
The diagram (right) shows how various chemicals, acting on the part of the hypothalamus that controls thirst and appetite, influence water and food intake under experiment conditions. In graph **A**, carbachol makes the subject most thirsty. In graph **B**, norepinephrine is most effective in producing hunger. All these chemicals occur naturally in the body and are monitored constantly by the hypothalamus.

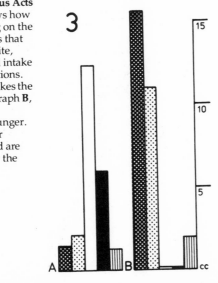

- ▨ Norepinephrine.
- ▒ Epinephrine.
- ☐ Carbachol.
- ■ Acetylcholine.
- ▥ NaCl.

4 Pituitary Hormones
When prompted by messages from the hypothalamus, the pituitary's two lobes (posterior, **A** and anterior, **B**) produce chemicals called hormones that enter the bloodstream and so find their way to the organs on which they must act.
The posterior lobe secretes two hormones:
a Oxytocin acts on a mother's womb after childbirth to make it contract and so lessen bleeding.
b Vasopressin is produced when high salt levels in the blood tell the hypothalamus that the body is low on water. Vasopressin acts on the kidneys and makes them reabsorb water that would otherwise be lost as urine.
The anterior lobe secretes

several hormones vital to body development:
c Adrenocorticotrophin (ACTH) acts on the adrenal glands over the kidneys, producing special hormones that help the body to withstand stress.
d, e Gonadotrophins act on the testes in men and the ovaries in women, producing further hormones vital for sexual development at adolescence, and menstruation in women.
f Thyrotrophin stimulates the thyroid gland to secrete hormones affecting the metabolic rate (the speed at which the body uses energy).
g Growth hormone, as its name suggests, controls the rate at which a child's body develops.
h Prolactin tells a new mother's breasts to produce milk.

©DIAGRAM

Fight or Flight Response

Arguably the most dramatic instance of the brain's rapid, widespread impact on the body is the so-called "fight or flight" response to sudden fear. A charging bull, a threatened mugging – such situations call forth a chain of bodily reactions triggered by the brain and designed to bring the body into readiness for sudden, violent activity. The sequence usually starts when the eyes see what the brain interprets as a threat. The idea of a threat sparks off fear or anger in one part of the brain and this provokes the hypothalamus to send a special signal to the pituitary gland's anterior (front) lobe. That lobe responds by pouring adrenocorticotrophic hormone (ACTH) out into the bloodstream.

Moments later this "stress" hormone invades the aptly named adrenal ("to-the-kidney") glands, one perched atop each kidney. Alerted in this fashion, the adrenals produce epinephrine and norepinephrine – two more stress-related hormones. The results are swift and all-pervasive. Briefly, the sympathetic nervous system triumphs over the parasympathetic nervous system. Organs needed for aggression or defense now get priority supplies of fuel and oxygen at the expense of organs routinely busying themselves with mere "civilian" affairs. What happens goes like this. Drastic changes affect the body's blood supply. The heart pumps harder and faster. Blood vessels that supply the skin and the digestive system contract, retarding the digestive process, and draining color from the skin. (If this is broken by an injury, blood escaping from the wound now readily coagulates.)

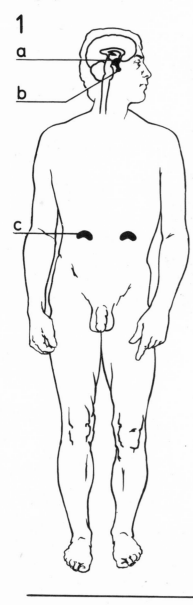

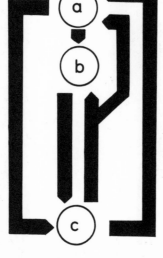

1 The Chemistry of Stress
The diagram (far left) shows the positions of organs primarily involved in the body's reaction to stress. Near left is a schematized diagram illustrating the flow of chemicals, their places of origin, and their target organs. The chain starts when the brain perceives a threat of some kind. The hypothalamus (a) then releases CRF, a chemical telling the pituitary (b) to secrete ACTH into the blood. When ACTH reaches the adrenal glands (c), the gland cortex produces corticoids that help the body cope with stress. While the body is under stress the medulla or center of the gland releases epinephrine. Hormone levels in the blood are monitored by (a) and (b).

At the same time, carbohydrate stored inside the liver is released as glucose that courses through the body in the blood, providing nourishment for brain and muscles.

Food must be combined with oxygen to yield the energy for fight or flight, so the chest expands, bronchial tubes widen, and breathing grows faster and deeper – all letting extra air into the lungs. Other changes happen just as quickly. Muscles tense, producing difficulty emptying rectum or bladder (though extreme terror may make that all too easy). Pupils of the eyes dilate. The mouth grows dry as its saliva output falls. The body sweats in readiness to cool itself in violent activity. Lastly, hair may stand on end – perhaps an evolutionary hangover from ancestors with potentially terrifying manes.

Scientists long ago traced back these events to ACTH released from the pituitary gland. But what triggered that release was a question baffling researchers for a generation. As one writer puts it, the task "consumed scores of research fellowships, hundreds of thousands of dollars, and millions of animals' brains."

In 1981 California's Salk Institute at last isolated the answer – a small molecule called CRF released by the hypothalamus in a stressed brain. But this discovery prompts new questions: for instance, are further chemical messengers involved, and can doctors find a use for CRF?

2 How Stress Affects the Body
The physical consequences of the hormonal preparation for fight or flight are dramatic. Epinephrine and norepinephrine act on many parts of the body, and the sympathetic nervous system readies the body for action. Among the resulting physical changes are:
a hair may stand on end;
b the pupils of the eyes dilate;
c saliva output falls;
d the skin pales as blood vessels supplying the skin contract;
e the chest expands as breathing becomes faster and deeper to deliver more oxygen to muscles;
f the heart beats faster and harder, and blood pressure rises;
g glucose is released from storage in the liver to provide food for muscles;
h digestion is slowed as the intestines' blood supply is partly rediverted;
i in extreme fear, bladder or rectum may empty;
j muscles tense, ready for fight or flight;
k if the skin is broken, blood coagulates more quickly;
l the body sweats, ready to cool itself if there is violent activity.

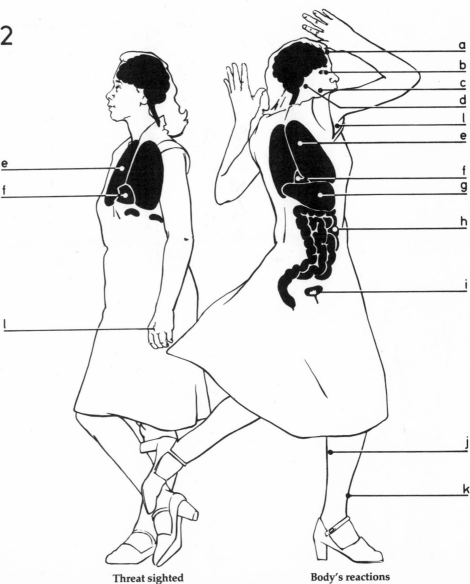

Threat sighted   Body's reactions

©DIAGRAM

Body Rhythms

Day by day, almost hour by hour, rhythms modify the workings of your brain and body.

Awake or asleep, the brain's activity runs in approximately 90-minute cycles, where relative tranquillity alternates with a frenzied eruption of electrical discharges to and from the brain's 10 billion cells. While you are awake, daydreaming succeeds periods when you feel mentally alert. In sleep, the rate of brain activity slows down, but even sleep has mental cycles too.

Daily rhythms affect much more than just the brain. Pulse rate, blood pressure, blood sugar level, body temperature, gland secretions, enzyme levels, salt secretion by the kidneys, intestinal contractions, cell growth – altogether more than 40 aspects of bodily activity routinely wax and wane

according to established patterns. This helps to explain why we feel lively, hungry, tired or maybe irritable at different times of day.

Biological changes of the kinds just mentioned are called circadian rhythms – rhythms that recur about once daily. Such cycles seem related to the Earth's daily revolution on its yearly path around the Sun. It is as if alarm clocks hidden in the body were programed to switch different bodily activities on and off at measured intervals in response to the great celestial cycle of day and night that dominates our lives. Indeed biologists call the mysterious controlling mechanisms biological clocks.

Many, if not all, circadian rhythms plainly benefit our bodies. For example, reduced urine flow at

1 Menstrual Rhythms

Ring **A** (right) illustrates the sequence of events in a woman's menstrual cycle, which is often, but not always, 28 days long. This body rhythm is governed by part of the hypothalamus and the pituitary – two closely linked areas in the brain which monitor and secrete hormones.

From about day 27 of the previous cycle, the pituitary produces FSH (follicle stimulating hormone, **a**) which makes a follicle in one of the ovaries begin to ripen an egg. Soon afterward, the follicle starts to secrete estrogen (**b**) – this hormone stimulates growth of the lining of the uterus (womb). A short burst of LH (luteinizing hormone, **c**) from the pituitary at about the midpoint of the cycle causes the follicle to release the egg and become a 'corpus luteum,' now secreting both estrogen and progesterone (**d**). The latter hormone prepares the lining of the uterus to receive a fertilized egg and stops LH production. If the egg is not fertilized, the corpus luteum shrinks and produces less estrogen and progesterone, so that the lining of the uterus eventually breaks down and carries away the egg – the process known as menstruation (**e**).

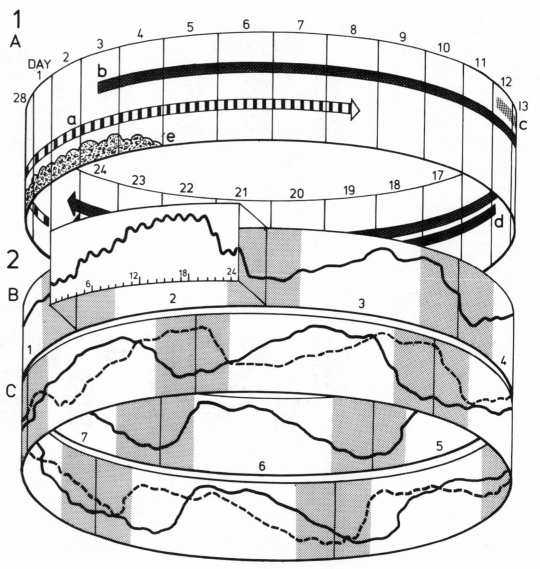

night helps to ensure a long spell of uninterrupted sleep, and regular sleep itself seems necessary to our health.

However, experiments have shown that within limits our body rhythms change if we are out of touch with the regular stimuli of day and night. Cavers, astronauts and others in perpetual light or dark find that their circadian rhythms tend to drift. Two groups of scientists in the unbroken daylight of an Arctic summer set their watches differently. Some adopted a 21-hour day; others a 27-hour day. Both sets found their body rhythms changed to fit the new regimes.

Experiments like this help to show how far biological clocks are inborn mechanisms, independent of the outer world. Whatever sets such clocks, they work in organisms too primitive to boast a brain. Yet there is no doubt that nerve impulses from some regions of the human brain do trigger regular activity. For instance, part of the hypothalamus controls a woman's monthly cycle. This works largely as a "feedback" process, triggered by estrogen hormone accumulating in the blood. But experiments with rats show that the hypothalamus acts only if the estrogen peaks in the afternoon; somehow the rat's hypothalamus is geared to the external rhythms produced by day and night.

Baboons – closer relatives to man than rats – show no such sensitivity. Yet scientists think the human hypothalamus is influenced by regions of the lower brain that help control body rhythms.

2 Circadian Rhythms

The two lower rings illustrate circadian, or daily rhythms. The upper ring (**B**), with its inset showing the 90-minute (ultradian) cycles, plots body temperature (the black line) and sleep periods (shaded areas) over a normal 24-hour day, seven-day week. The lower ring (**C**) is a graph based on measurements of a man adapting to an artificial 28-hour day, 6-day week in a cave. This man adapted well to a longer day, his body temperature falling as it should during each 9-hour sleep period. His companion's body, however, continued in its 24-hour cycle (shown by the broken line), resulting in disturbed sleep. Most people are unable to tolerate a 28-hour circadian rhythm – the ability to adapt quickly and successfully to a longer or shorter 'day' is a useful attribute for such people as astronauts.

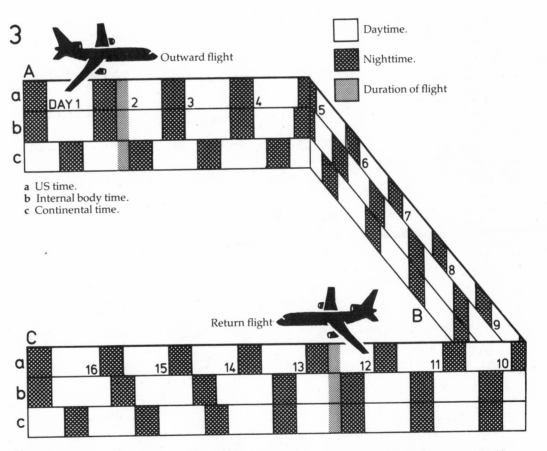

a US time.
b Internal body time.
c Continental time.

Daytime.

Nighttime.

Duration of flight.

3 Upsetting the Body's Clock

Jet lag is a common example of the effects of altering the body's internal clock. A return journey to Europe by air means that the clock is desynchronized twice, producing strain on the body and temporarily reducing mental capability. At the start, (**A**), the body is adjusted to US time, but after the outward flight on Day 2 that time zone no longer applies and the traveler finds that he is wakeful at night and sleepy by day. It takes about a week for the rhythm to adjust (**B**) to new local time. On return, the body clock is upset again and does not reset itself properly for another three or four days (**C**).

©DIAGRAM

Sleeping and Dreaming

Each night we switch off conscious, rational thought, and switch on streams of zany mental images. An average person spends 20 years of life asleep, experiencing at least 300,000 dreams. Plainly, sleep and dreams matter to us, though people have survived years with little sleep. But until recently scientists had few clues to how sleep works or why. Now we have begun to grasp its mechanisms and its roles.

Like consciousness, sleep is an active process of the nervous system. When darkness falls, the eyes indirectly inform a biological clock – the pineal gland deep inside the brain. The pineal gland then yields melatonin – a hormone that affects brain cells which use serotonin. This is a sleep-related chemical transmitter concentrated in the raphe nuclei aligned along the brainstem behind the reticular activating system – the part responsible for consciousness.

In sleep, sensory input to this last system is reduced and the electrical activity sweeping from it up through the cerebral cortex drops below the level required to keep the individual awake. Yet a sleeping person's brain by no means switches off. Sleep involves repeated cycles of activity, each marked by several stages. In Stage One, the individual relaxes and drifts in and out of sleep. In Stage Two, the eyes start to roll slowly from side to side. The slightest noise may jerk the individual awake. In Stage Three, the body grows still more relaxed, and a loud noise would be needed to rouse the sleeper. Twenty minutes after sleep began, the

1 Sleep Centers in Brainstem
The diagram (below) shows the location of areas in the brainstem associated with sleep. The locus coeruleus (**a**) is a small patch of dark cells which is thought to produce a secretion initiating REM sleep, in which we dream. The raphe nuclei (**b**) are nuclei within the reticular formation of the brainstem that secrete a substance which acts on the formation to produce light sleep. The reticular formation as a whole (**c**) normally acts to keep us awake and alert – even while we sleep it is watchful and ready to rouse us should the need arise.

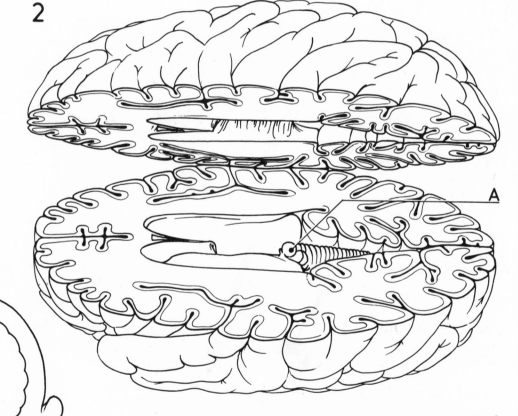

2 The Pineal Gland
The diagram (above) shows the brain split in two, horizontally, to reveal the pineal gland – a tiny structure (**A**) at the top of the brainstem. The two thalami have been removed to show the pineal gland more clearly. The gland seems to act as a little clock within the brain, keeping track of the body's natural cycles and registering external factors like light and darkness. A chemical it secretes starts the chain of events leading to sleep.

deep sleep of Stage Four sets in. Then the cycle shifts into reverse: back through stages Three and Two.

Instead of exactly re-experiencing Stage One, the sleeper enters the first of several phases of so-called paradoxical or rapid-eye-movement sleep (REM for short). In this stage noradrenalin-producing cells in the pons – the middle section of the brainstem – fire off a battery of signals that spread to nearby cells and then affect the cerebral cortex. According to the activation-synthesis theory, the cortex draws on "memory banks" to help to build a pattern from these signals, and the bizarre result is what we call a dream. Meanwhile the eyes rapidly shift to and fro beneath closed lids as they scan dream images created in the mind. At the same time signals from the brain paralyze the large muscles, so preventing violent movements of the limbs.

Each sleep cycle lasts some 90 minutes, and most people experience four or five cycles per night. The need for sleep and dreams can be explained in several ways. Deep sleep stimulates growth hormone that builds and repairs body tissues. REM sleep conceivably restores the weary brain. In Freudian psychoanalysis, dreaming (incidentally not all of it confined to REM sleep) expresses repressed sexual desires. More modern thinking favors dreams as harmonizing the sleeper's inner world with his environment; rehearsing genetic patterns of behavior; or helping the mind sort and file the day's experiences.

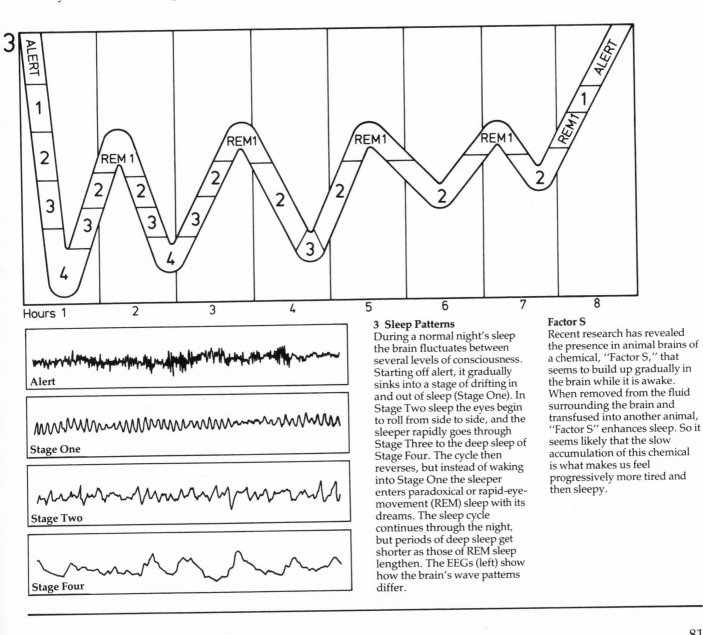

3 Sleep Patterns
During a normal night's sleep the brain fluctuates between several levels of consciousness. Starting off alert, it gradually sinks into a stage of drifting in and out of sleep (Stage One). In Stage Two sleep the eyes begin to roll from side to side, and the sleeper rapidly goes through Stage Three to the deep sleep of Stage Four. The cycle then reverses, but instead of waking into Stage One the sleeper enters paradoxical or rapid-eye-movement (REM) sleep with its dreams. The sleep cycle continues through the night, but periods of deep sleep get shorter as those of REM sleep lengthen. The EEGs (left) show how the brain's wave patterns differ.

Factor S
Recent research has revealed the presence in animal brains of a chemical, "Factor S," that seems to build up gradually in the brain while it is awake. When removed from the fluid surrounding the brain and transfused into another animal, "Factor S" enhances sleep. So it seems likely that the slow accumulation of this chemical is what makes us feel progressively more tired and then sleepy.

© DIAGRAM

The Emotions

The brain "feels" as well as thinks. We need our emotions. Properly balanced by reason, they help us to react appropriately to the people and objects with which we share our world. They also help us to draw wished for responses from others. Emotions forge bonds between the infant and her mother; the husband and his wife. A good guide to the importance to us of emotions is the human face, which can produce more expressions to reflect its moods than that of any other animal. Even changes in the sizes of pupils of the eyes offer subtle visual clues to how one person reacts to another.

The brain mechanisms that produce emotions have been partly mapped since 1953. That year, Canadian scientists discovered that a rat gained intense pleasure when a tiny electrical current was passed via a microelectrode through part of the hypothalamus deep inside its brain. Some rats pressed a treadle for 24 hours nonstop to keep current exciting this brain pleasure center. Researchers also found that the hypothalamus holds so-called aversion centers. Exciting these made rats act as though scared or suffering pain. Experiments with animals and brain-damaged people have betrayed other centers of emotion. Most lie in the limbic system that envelops the top of the brainstem. Stimulating an amygdala above the hypothalamus may spark off reactions of rage and aggression. Removing the same mass of nerves altogether made an infuriated epileptic childlike and docile. Stimulating the nearby septum may cheer up severely depressed individuals. However, a slight shift in the stimulus

Centers of Emotion
Most of the centers of human emotion are located in the limbic system at the top of the brainstem (located on the diagram near right), and in the hypothalamus. Stimulating these centers in different sites and with different intensities of stimulus produces variations in an individual's emotional responses.
1 This diagram shows the emotional centers located in the limbic system.
a Septum pellucidum.
b Hippocampus.
c Amygdala.

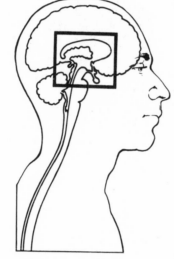

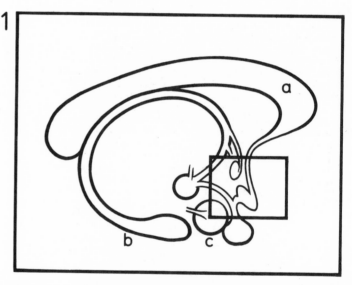

2 Hypothalamic Centers
The two main areas in the hypothalamus associated with emotions are the dorsomedial nucleus, which controls aggressive behavior and emotions, and the dorsal area, which is thought to be the human "pleasure site."
A Dorsomedial nucleus.
B Dorsal area.

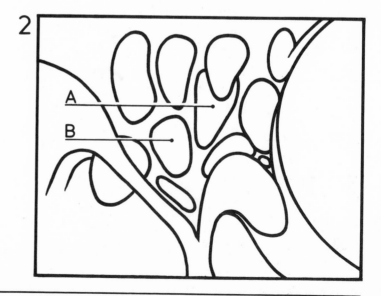

produces various results. Exciting the amygdala, septum or hippocampus in different places may make people agitated, anxious, elated, excited or enraged.

Scientists remain unsure just how the brain's emotional mechanism works. Most likely the cerebral cortex tells the limbic system the kind of response to make, and the limbic system adjusts the response level, from mild enjoyment to ecstacy, or from vague displeasure to intense hatred. Changes in the flow and take-up of neurotransmitters in brain cells directly produce changes in emotion. Pleasurable sensations may be linked with chemical signals produced by the release of noradrenalin, while pain unleashes extra acetylcholine. Mood state seems geared to the chemical serotonin, lack of which makes people feel depressed.

An emotional experience plainly involves feedback via sensory nerves to the brain from internal glands and organs. Conversely, changes in the brain affect internal glands and organs in ways that lead to an emotional experience. This brain-body link is the basis of the lie-detector, a device recording changes in the electrical property of skin produced by altered sweat-gland activity.

The emotionally stressed brain can even act upon the body to produce a gastric ulcer.

The emotional level at which your limbic system operates helps to determine how you perceive reality. This is largely why some people sense pain more readily than others, and why a scene that depresses one individual exhilarates another.

3 Expression
Facial expression is a means of both displaying and conveying emotion. Subtle variations in the expression are the results of minute movements of the facial muscles. Although many facial expressions can be assumed at will, many more are involuntary reactions to pleasant or unpleasant stimuli, and instantly convey our emotional reactions. The illustrations below show a variety of facial expressions, including pleasure, disgust, surprise, fear, pain and disapproval.

4 Pupil Enlargement
In the 1960s Eckhard Hess of the University of Chicago noted that when a person is excited or interested, or otherwise stimulated, the pupils of the eyes enlarge. By instinct or association, enlarged pupils then make the person affected more attractive to the opposite sex – not because enlarged pupils are more esthetically pleasing, but because the reaction displays interest and stimulation. Consequently many people, when shown pictures that are identical except for pupil size, will find the picture depicting the larger pupils (**b**) more attractive than that showing normal-sized pupils (**a**).

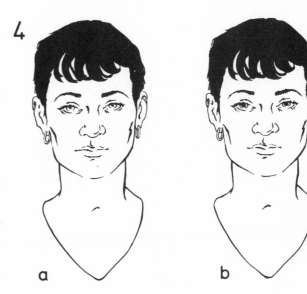

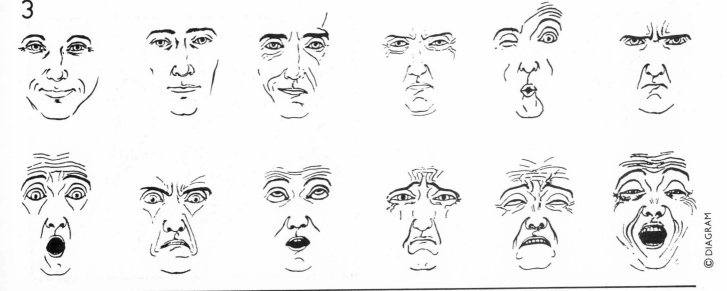

Sex and Sexuality

Directly and indirectly, the brain is deeply involved with sexual emotions, and indeed with sexuality itself.

In both sexes, sex drive and response seem to be sparked off by events occurring in the sense organs or hypothalamus. Stimulating laboratory animals with microelectrodes implanted in the front part of this structure makes males ejaculate and females grow receptive to males. In human beings, damage to the same part of the brain impairs sexual function.

Hypothalamus and limbic system are both genetically programed for patterns of instinctive sexual behavior, but this is largely triggered by sex hormones latching onto receptor sites in the brain's hypothalamus, amygdala and other centers of the old, inner brain.

Research suggests that the brain's exposure to sex hormones at a critical phase in very early life determines sexual behavior for the rest of life, irrespective of an individual's apparent sex. In rats, females briefly given male hormones for a few days just after birth fail to mate as females should and cannot ovulate. Significantly, the preoptic part of their hypothalami shows characteristically male, not female, neuron patterns. Girls born with too much male hormone behave like boys, showing little interest in playing the normal girlish game of "being mother."

The brain's influence on sexuality affects many aspects of our lives. For instance, female hormones reduce the level in the brain of chemicals called monoamine oxidase inhibitors. People with low levels of these substances are highly arousable.

1 Sex roles

As investigation into the brain's activities advances, the processes which make a person male or female are seen to be more and more complex.
A child's "basic" sex is determined at conception by the X or Y chromosome carried by the fertilizing sperm. A hormonal chain reaction is then active in the developing fetus, producing characteristically male or female genitals and gonads. Apart from the genitals, body appearance is virtually identical in pre-puberty males and females (**A**) until hormonal activity at puberty makes the adult sex differences more overt (**B**).

However, research is increasingly suggesting that hormonal activity around birth produces physiological differences in the brains of males and females; these differences are thought to be responsible for girls' gentle, motherly interests and boys' more aggressive traits. Natural or artificially induced hormone imbalance can produce "male" changes in female brains and vice versa, and related personality changes – girls exhibit more aggression, boys become gentler. These results suggest that sex roles may be as much a result of brain development as of social conditioning.

1

A   B

Supposedly this explains why women are generally held to be more easily alarmed, stressed or otherwise aroused than men.

Women are particularly liable to emotional upset just before they menstruate. Many grow depressed and irritable as hormones "hit" the brain. They are four times likelier to commit crime now than earlier or later in their monthly cycle. (Incidentally, the contraceptive pills that tamper with the cycle deceive the brain to do so.) Difference in brain function between the sexes helps explain why women tend to be more sensitive than men to taste, touch and loud sounds, and why men react faster yet are more readily distracted by novelty. At least some differences between the sexes seem to stem from how they use each half of the brain (see page 108).

Maybe even brain structure is involved. In both sexes a part of the top of one temporal lobe is larger than the matching part in the other temporal lobe, but this difference is more marked in men.

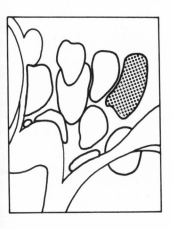

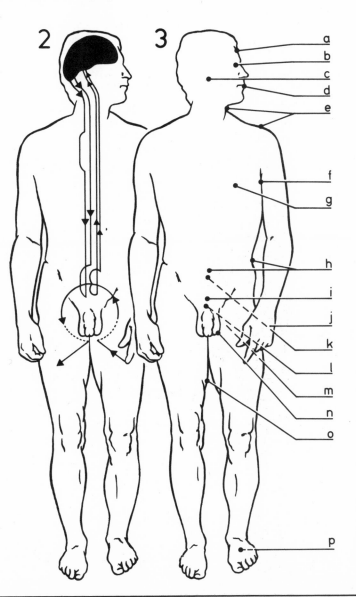

2 Sex Drive
Sex drive is made up of three components: genetically programed sexual behavior patterns; the activity of sex hormones; and an individual's response to environmental stimuli. All of these components are controlled in males and females by a site known as the posterior hypothalamic area, located in the hypothalamus as shown above. Response to a sexual stimulus is a reflex action along a pathway (shown right) involving nerve fibers in the brain, the spinal column and the genitals.

3 Erogenous Zones
Numerous areas in the male and female body are capable of producing sexual arousal when stimulated. The major erogenous zones are listed here.
a Scalp.
b Eyelids.
c Ears.
d Mouth and tongue.
e Neck and shoulders.
f Insides of arms.
g Breasts and nipples.
h Waist and navel.
i Abdomen.
j Hands.
k Small of back.
l Base of spine.
m Buttocks.
n Genitals.
o Insides of thighs.
p Soles of feet.

© DIAGRAM

Personality

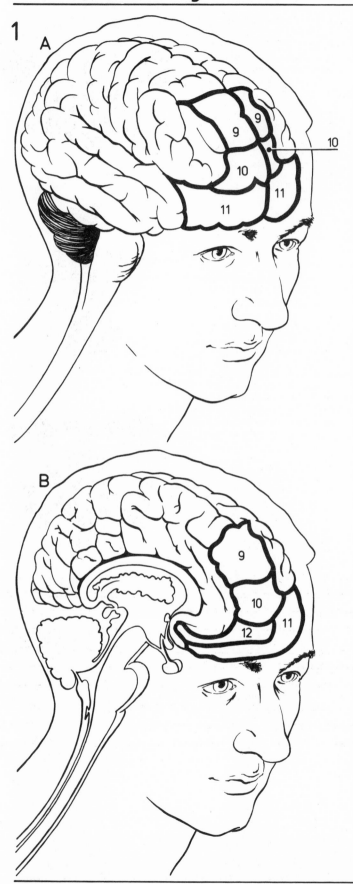

One afternoon in 1848 a railroad construction company foreman called Phineas Gage poured some gunpowder into a narrow hole in a rock. Then he tamped down the gunpowder with a long, heavy metal rod. Unluckily a spark set off the charge and drove the rod clean through his skull, damaging the brain just behind his forehead. Amazingly, he lived, with powers of memory and thought apparently intact. Yet the mild-spoken, efficient foreman had become foul mouthed, bad tempered and erratic. Damage to the frontal lobes – those with the largest, least understood areas of cerebral cortex – had drastically changed Gage's personality.

Defined by one writer as "that mixture of emotional character and thought," personality seemingly involves more than just the frontal lobes, as patients suffering epileptic seizures reveal. Those with an affected right temporal lobe tend to be emotionally responsive, concerned for detail, helpless and sexually oriented. Patients suffering a left temporal lobe epileptic focus tend to be religious, moralistic, inflexible, sober and self deprecating.

Evidently personality involves interaction between large areas of cortex and the limbic system – that older, inner emotional brain.

Lack of knowledge of brain mechanisms has not stopped mindwatchers coming up with theories to explain personality. The Austrian psychoanalyst, Sigmund Freud, theorized that personality develops as children pass through five stages involving interest in specific parts of the body and

1 The Prefrontal Cortex
The Brodmann areas 9 through 12 make up the prefrontal cortex, shown (**A**) on the complete human brain and on a median cross-section (**B**). The prefrontal cortex is responsible for an individual's responses to circumstances; these responses may range from despair, anxiety and dislike to ecstasy, optimism and delight. The prefrontal cortex is not involved with intellect, but with emotional response; damage or surgery affecting the area will tend to make a person more passive, with lesser extremes of emotional response.

named by Freud oral, anal, phallic, latent, and genital. Freud thought that problems encountered at any stage fixated an individual at that stage. He also believed that each individual's personality involved a tug-of-war between three components: the selfish, pleasure-seeking, amoral *id*, the moral perfectionist *superego* (the conscience), and the *ego*, a realist which seeks a balance.

Freud's influential successors included Alfred Adler, who argued for self-imposed goals and social relationships as influences on personality; and Carl Gustav Jung, who developed the idea of personality complexes: with shy, introverted people at one end of a personality scale and outgoing, extraverted individuals at the other. Refining this idea, Professor Hans Eysenck has suggested that inhibitory brain-cell signals outnumber excitatory signals in introverts, while in extraverts the imbalance is the other way. Personality assessment plays a useful part in assessing mental patients and applicants for responsible positions. Psychologists may use any of a battery of tests. Some measure personality according to a given scale. For instance, the 16PF test devised by the American psychologist R.B. Cattell takes account of 16 personality traits. Eysenck tests for tendency to introversion or extraversion, and stability or neuroticism. So-called projective tests are less precise but may be more revealing. They involve the subject's responses to meaningless or ambiguous stimuli as guides to how his mind is working.

2 Rorschach Ink Blots
The Swiss psychiatrist Herman Rorschach felt that a person's response to a random image illustrates factors affecting their personality. Rorschach showed his test subjects ten different ink blots, some colored and some black and white, and asked the subjects to relate images and ideas provoked by each blot. With tests such as these there is no "right" or "wrong" answer, but the results may help to provide clues to a person's personality traits or temporary state of mind.

3 Development of Emotion
The mature human is able to experience and recognize a wide variety of emotional responses. This capacity is not present at birth, but is developed through prematurity by an increased experience of emotional stimuli coinciding with the brain's development. One theory on early emotional development considers that newborn infants originally experience only a generalized sensation of excitement, which soon polarizes into pleasure or distress. As the child matures, these two sensations branch into the more subtle distinctions of the emotions as we know them; the more subtle the distinction between emotions, the later a child experiences them.

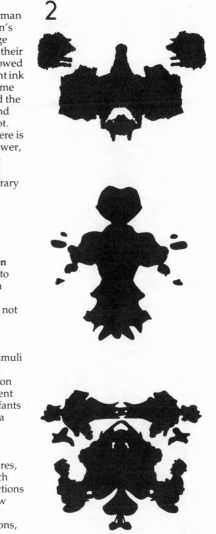

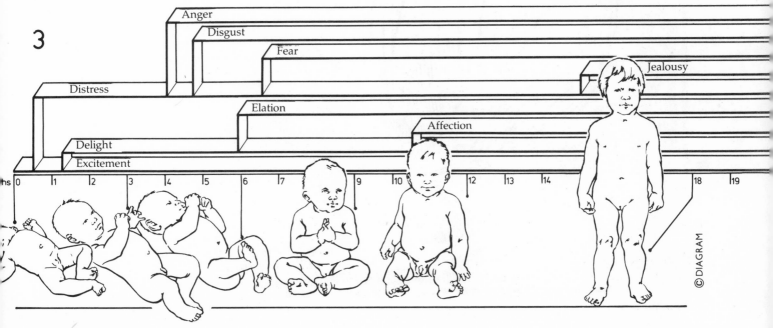

©DIAGRAM

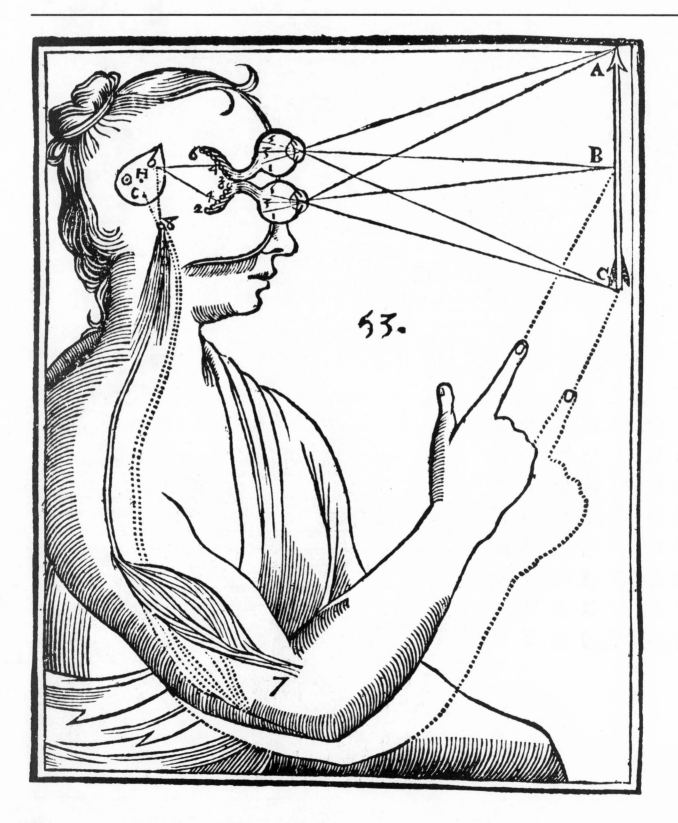

Chapter 6

AWARENESS AND THOUGHT

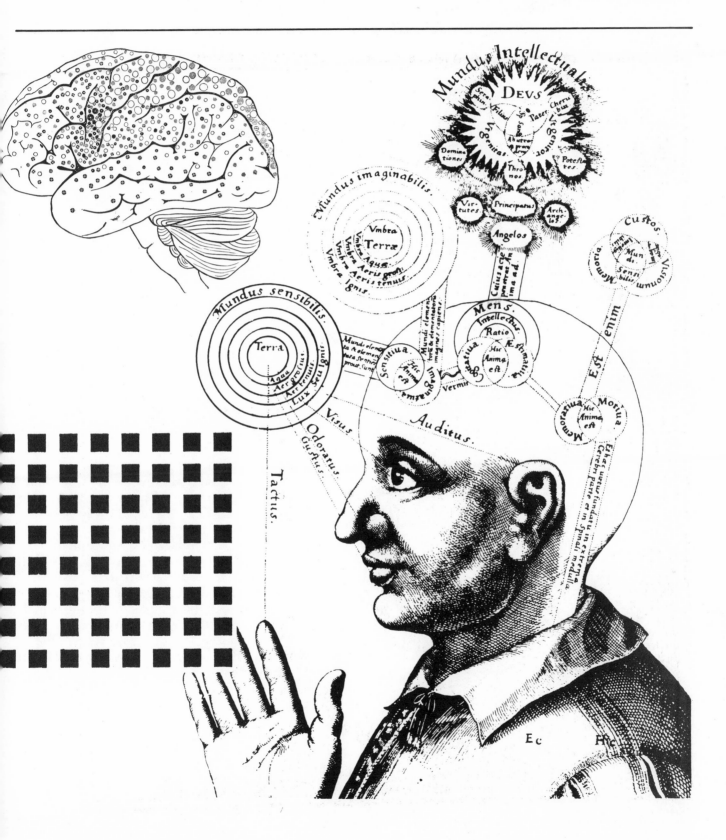

Controlling Movements

1 **A**

B

C

2

A Jaw and tongue.
B Lips.
C Face.
D Fingers.
E Hand.
F Arm.
G Trunk.
H Leg.

2 Motor and Premotor Cortex
Each cerebral hemisphere has a
strip of cortex (**a**) that initiates
muscular action (motor cortex).
In front of it is another strip (**b**)
which controls it, planning its
actions in the light of past
experience (premotor cortex).
Diagrams show the location of
these two strips (right), and
(above) which parts of the
motor cortex control body parts.
Comparatively large areas deal
with movements of lips and
hands.

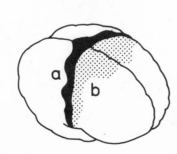

1 Central Nervous System
Seven subsystems in the central
nervous system control
movement.
A Spinal reflexes act rapidly to
protect the body from harm.
Incoming signals from skin,
muscles and joints do not have
to be fed to the brain, so
response time is shortened.

B Vestibular nuclei in the pons
(**a**) and cerebellum (**b**) help us
keep our balance. Posture is also
aided by a pathway from the
midbrain tectum (**c**) which
relates posture to signals from
eyes and ears.
C Commands originated in the
motor cortex (**d**) are relayed to
muscles controlling postural
adjustment by the reticular
formation in the brainstem (**e**).

The pioneer English neurologist Hughlings
Jackson once claimed that movement is the main
task of the nervous system. This seems believable
when we consider the bewildering array of brain
structures controlling muscle action.
Immediate control of muscles comes from motor
neurons arising in the spinal cord and brainstem,
and making muscles contract or relax, so switching
movements on and off. Cell bodies of the spinal
motor neurons lie in the gray matter of the spinal
cord. Cell bodies of the brainstem occur as nuclei:
roots of cranial nerves operating muscles in the
head and face. Each muscle fiber is operated by an
on-off mechanism, but complex nerve pathways
between controlling motor systems in the brain
trigger and inhibit activity by sets of muscles in
sequences that make coordinated movements
possible and prevent opposing muscles acting
simultaneously, for that would paralyze the limbs
that they control.
The central nervous system has no fewer than
seven subsystems devoted to controlling

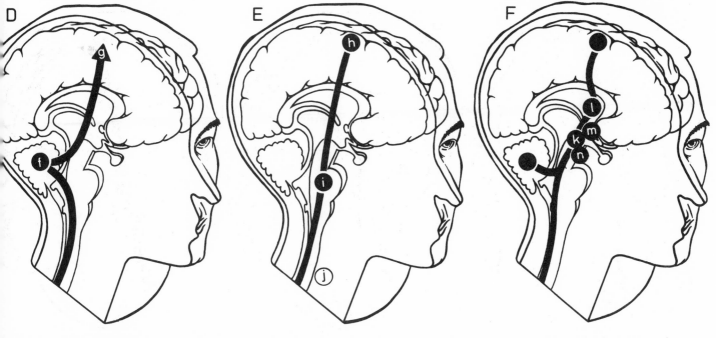

D The cerebellum (**f**) influences motor systems in the brainstem and also the motor cortex in the cerebrum (**g**). The cerebellum modifies signals to help control direction, rate, force and steadiness of quick intentional movements.

E The pyramidal tracts are two pathways which link the cerebral cortex (**h**) directly with the brainstem (**i**) and spinal cord (**j**). These pathways help to control skilled, coordinated movements requiring training, for example playing the violin.

F The extrapyramidal system consists of pathways which ensure smoothly continuous movements of limbs, especially hands and arms. They also halt movement. Several parts of the central nervous system are involved in the extrapyramidal system, including:

k Parts of the thalamus.
l The basal ganglia.
m The brainstem's red nucleus.
n The substantia nigra. Pathways from the cerebellum and cerebral cortex are also involved.

movement.
1 Spinal reflex pathways automatically respond to incoming signals from skin, muscles and joints to adjust posture and pull limbs away from painful stimuli like thorns or scalding water.
2 Vestibular nuclei in the brainstem's pons and a nearby "old" inner region of the cerebellum work to help us keep our balance.
3 A pathway from the midbrain's tectum ("roof") seemingly helps to relate posture to signals received from the ears and eyes.
4 Obeying commands from the cerebral cortex, descending pathways inside the brainstem's reticular formation send forth powerful "act" or "don't act" instructions to the muscles that control postural adjustment.
5 The cerebellum strongly influences motor systems in the brainstem and the part of the cerebral cortex that sends out motor signals. The cerebellum helps to control direction, rate, force and steadiness of quick intentional movements.
6 Two pathways link cerebral cortex directly with

brainstem and spinal cord. Named pyramidal tracts, because they form the medulla's pyramidal bulges, these pathways help to control precise, skilled movements requiring training: for instance playing the violin, or hurdling.
7 Nearby pathways making up the extrapyramidal system appear to assure smoothly continuous movements of the limbs, especially the hands and arms. They also bring movement to a halt. This complicated group of brain structures includes parts of the thalamus, the basal ganglia, the red nucleus and substantia nigra in the brainstem, pathways from the cerebellum, and certain others from the cerebral cortex.
Particular actions are triggered by signals fired from a specific region of a motor strip on the cerebrum. In turn motor signals stem from orders that the motor strip received from the nearby sensory strip, but via the thalamus. However, the will to make a muscle move probably arises in the brain's frontal lobes.

©DIAGRAM

Consciousness

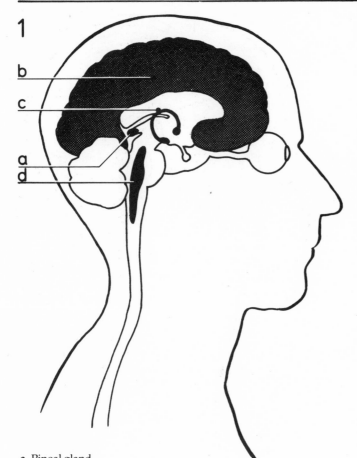

a Pineal gland.
b Cerebrum.
c Limbic system.
d Reticular formation.

1 The Seat of Consciousness
Consciousness is so vital a brain function that men have been anxious to determine its location, leading to several inaccurate early ideas.
a René Descartes, seventeenth-century French philosopher, believed consciousness was located in the pineal gland at the top of the brainstem.
b Neurologists early this century claimed it was to be found in the cerebrum.
c Later opinion said it lay in the limbic system.
d It now seems likely that consciousness is a function of the reticular formation, a network of cells in the oldest part of the brain – the brainstem.

People disagree about what consciousness implies. Some equate consciousness with self-awareness. Many think of consciousness as the activity of the mind, something supposedly more than just a function of the brain. One scientist simply and precisely defines consciousness as the activity of all neurons not otherwise engaged, multiplied by their connections.

Without consciousness the body functions little better than a cabbage. People sought the seat of consciousness for centuries. The seventeenth-century French philosopher René Descartes located consciousness in the pineal gland. Early this century neurologists placed it in the convoluted cerebrum, acclaimed then as center of our highest faculties. From there, academic theory moved it to the limbic system. Research suggests that consciousness resides in none of these, but in the reticular formation, a group of cells inside the brainstem – oldest, "lowliest" region of the brain.

Besides their main paths to the cerebral cortex, sensory nerves route branch lines through the recticular formation. Many of its cells supply the thalamus. From there, other cells fan out around the brain: to hypothalamus, corpus striatum, cerebellum, and different regions of the cerebral cortex. Various kinds of stimuli fed in to the brain start the reticular formation firing signals at targets all around the brain, measurably altering electrical impulses from the cerebral cortex and arousing this so-called higher center.

As one writer puts it, the cerebral cortex without the reticular formation to drive it is like a great computer without a power supply.

Without the reticular formation's alerting signals the brain grows sleepy. Damage to this same arousing mechanism can cause unconsciousness. Irreversible damage produces coma, and sometimes death. Indeed irretrievable loss of consciousness is an important criterion employed for judging if a patient is clinically dead.

Yet "consciousness" is not quite as simple as all this suggests. For instance, consciousness has different levels through which you pass when you awaken from sleep or general anesthetic, as your reticular formation accelerates the brain waves coursing through your cerebral cortex.

Even wide wake, we are not equally aware of all the influences or activities inside our brain. For instance, we may experience unconscious (that is, subconscious) thoughts. Then, too, practiced drivers change gears "unconsciously."

2

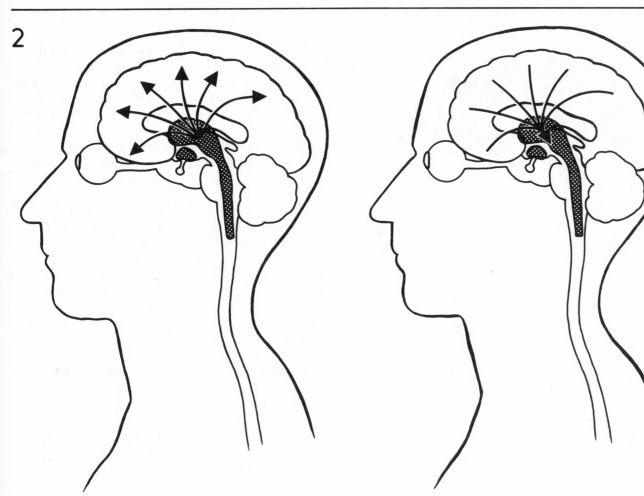

2 The Reticular Formation at Work

The diagram (above left) shows how the reticular formation, acting on information supplied to it, sends out signals at targets around the brain. In this way it sustains or increases electrical activity in the cerebral cortex. The diagram (above right) shows how pathways carrying commands from the higher regions of the brain link up with incoming sensory signals in the brainstem to keep the reticular formation informed of events.

3A

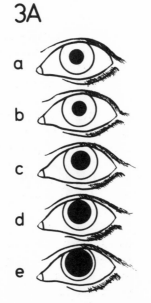

a

b

c

d

e

3 Levels of Consciousness

A Pupil size is one of the criteria used by anesthetists to gauge the level of consciousness of a patient. Diagram **a** is the pupil of a patient using painkillers whose consciousness is unaffected. Pupil **b** looks similar, and shows light anesthesia. However **c, d** and **e** show progressively deepening anesthesia with corresponding increase in pupil size.

B EEG recordings are a useful guide to state of consciousness and help to tell when brain death may have occurred. The second trace from top shows the regular pattern of alpha waves in relaxation (eyes closed).

3B

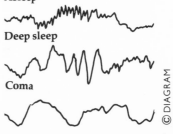

Excited

Relaxed

Drowsy

Asleep

Deep sleep

Coma

©DIAGRAM

Attention and Habituation

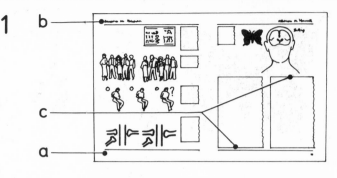

1 Selectivity by Training
When you turned to the page, did you notice: **a** that the page numbers are upside down; **b** that the heading is in a different typeface; **c** that a line of text has been printed twice?
Chances are that you did not because your attention mechanism does not consider them important. However, a proofreader with trained selective vision would have noticed these errors very quickly.

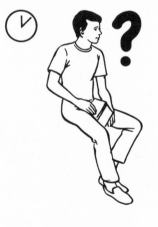

2 Selectivity by Sex
Sex conditions the way we see things and what we pay attention to. Shaded areas in each group of figures on the left indicate what a woman (far left) might notice and what a man (left) might pay attention to.

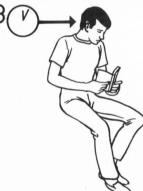
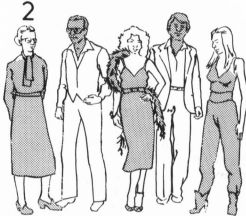

3 Selective Screening
Ten to 15 repetitions of a stimulus at one second intervals are enough to stop response by neurons in the reticular formation. This is why we cease to hear the regular ticking of a clock after a while. However, if the clock stops, the brain may register the novelty of the ensuing silence.

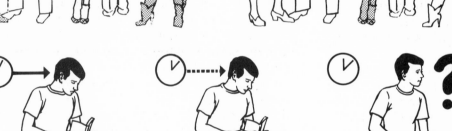
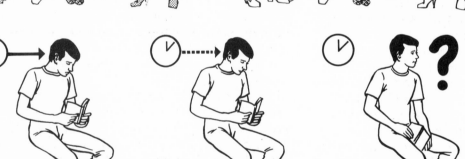
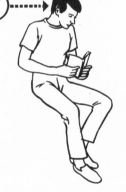
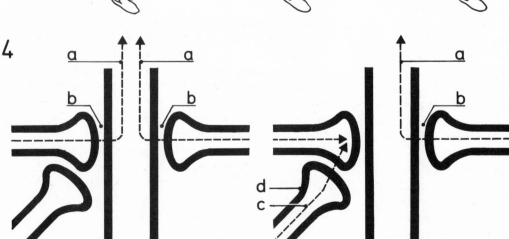

4 How Habituation Works
When signals recording a new stimulus (**a**) make their way to the brain, chemicals called neurotransmitters allow the impulses to jump across gaps (synapses) (**b**), unimpeded. However, when the stimulus is regularly repeated other neurotransmitters (**c**) are released by a modifying neuron (**d**). These inhibit the passage of signals across the synapse and cut down the flow of impulses to the brain.

5 Left and Right Thalamus
Part of the selective attention mechanism of the brain lies in the thalami. Experimental evidence shows that the left thalamus helps us to pay attention to phenomena which can be translated into words, while the right thalamus helps us to concentrate on visual images.

5

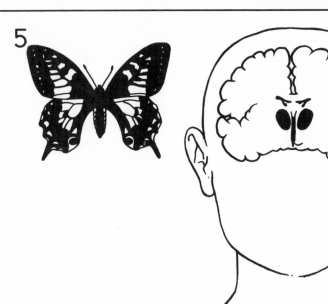

butterfly

The famous Canadian neurosurgeon Wilder Penfield once said that, granted a second life, he would have spent it studying the mechanism of the brain that makes it possible for us to focus our attention on one concept at a time. This faculty of selective consciousness determines what we do from one instant to another.

Penfield surmised that when we concentrate upon a particular matter, the "highest brain mechanism" has the brain's sensory-motor mechanism shut out the inflow of all other information but let related memories reach consciousness. He reasoned that selecting what enters the stream of consciousness is a subconscious activity of the brain's automatic sensory-motor mechanism, for he knew victims of epileptic automatism can walk home unaware.

The English psychologist Donald Broadbent also argued persuasively for selective filters in the brain turning out all incoming signals but the one we want to receive.

Experiments at Oxford in the 1960s threw some light upon selective attention. Subjects listening to two different voices simultaneously via earphones were told to concentrate on one ear only. They recalled little from the other ear except a change of voice or language, or the mention of their name. This ability subconsciously to monitor seemingly disregarded stimuli gained the apt name of "cocktail party phenomenon" from the fact that mention of your own name seems to stand out above general party babble. The same attention phenomenon occurs when a baby's muffled cry wakens its mother sleeping in a noisy room or

wakens its mother sleeping in a noisy room or produces changes in her heartbeat, skin resistance and brainwave pattern.

At least part of the brain's selective attention mechanism evidently lies inside the two thalami. Experiments and studies with brain-damaged patients show that the left thalamus helps us to pay attention to things around us describable in words, while the right thalamus helps us to pay attention to visual shapes.

Malfunction of part of the selective attention mechanism may help to explain why some otherwise mentally normal children have certain learning difficulties; why autistic children live turned in on their inner worlds; why schizophrenics tend to confuse their inner world with outer reality. This theory, though, remains unproved.

Intriguingly, microelectrodes implanted in brains reveal so-called novelty-recording cells that fire only in response to a new stimulus. Ten to 15 repetitions at one second intervals are enough to stop response by neurons in the brainstem's reticular formation – the area involved with general arousal. This shows why we immediately notice when a neighbor begins to mow his lawn, but soon lose awareness of the mower's noise.

When this happens we say we are habituated to the sound. Of course, neurons stop firing when they get fatigued, but, unlike these, habituated neurons can be reactivated by a strong, sudden stimulus like a loud sound or a flash of light.

©DIAGRAM

Perception: 1

Some brain-damaged people can see but not perceive: their eyes work normally but the brain is unaware of signals from the eyes because the brain cells that process visual information have been damaged. These people suffer a great disadvantage, for most of what the brain perceives depends on information from the eyes, and perception is essential to thought and judgment. Indeed, one writer calls perception unconscious thought.

How we perceive the world around us depends on several factors – some inborn, some learned. The inborn tendency of nerve cells to tire and give false readings can make the same thing appear quite different to us at different times. You can prove this by staring at special drawings showing parallel slanting lines, then at drawings showing parallel vertical lines. Brain cells that registered the slanting lines have tired more than cells registering lines at other angles. The effect is to make the vertical lines appear to slant the other way. Similarly, when you stop a flat spiral shape rotating on a record turntable, the spiral seems to go on rotating but in the opposite direction. This is probably because the brain cells detecting movement in the first direction have tired and stopped their rapid firing, so that you become aware of the normal random firings from the brain cells that detect movement in the opposite direction.

In the same way how hot or cold a bowl of water feels depends partly upon how long your hands have been immersed, and thus how tired are the neurons that register heat and cold. As a last

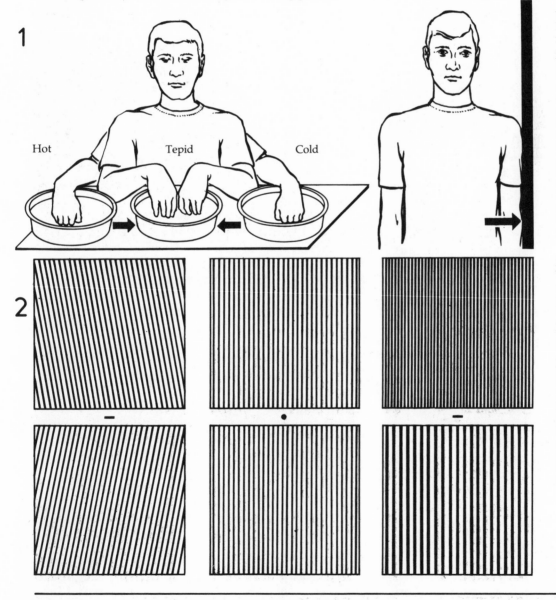

1

Hot   Tepid   Cold

2

1 Fooling the Brain
If sensory nerves send messages to the brain saying the same thing for a long time, the brain cells eventually become tired, and when the stimulus stops, the cells registering opposite sensations influence our perception. For example, hands immersed in hot or cold water for a while think that tepid water is either colder or hotter than it really is (far left). In the same way, if you press against a wall as shown (near left), when you stand clear your arm will feel very light, and may even rise up, because it previously felt so heavy.

2 Visual Tricks
These games show how the nerves registering visual information rapidly become habituated. Focus your eyes for one minute on the short line between the squares on the far left, moving your gaze from one end of the line to the other. Then look at the dot between the center pair of squares. What happens to the center squares? Focus for one minute on the short line between the right-hand pair of squares, again shifting your gaze from one end to the other. Move back to the center dot. What happens to the center squares now?

example, pressing your arm against a wall can affect how heavy you perceive your arm to be. As intriguing as the effects of nerve-cell fatigue on perception is the brain's seemingly inborn tendency to organize things seen into patterns. Thus after a while, the small black squares that make up a visual grid seem to form regular groups. "Proximity" is psychology's name for the effect whereby we perceive a grid of dots as made up of vertical rows if the horizontal gaps between dots are greater than the vertical ones. "Similarity" describes the effect where we see equally spaced dots as vertical columns if each vertical row differs in color from the next.

In the early 1900s so-called Gestalt ("form") psychologists used such examples to suggest that the brain contains electrical fields that tend to perceive simple shapes; but modern research favors an explanation of perception as the brain coordinating different specialized nerve cells to accept, reject and modify data received. This suggests that learning plays a large part in perception. The next pages explore this idea.

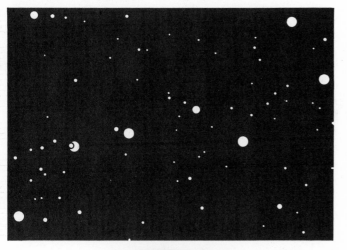

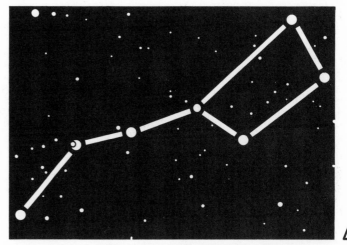

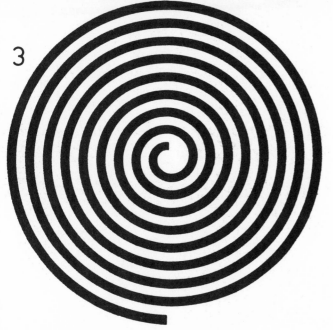

3 Motion
Make a copy of the spiral shape on the left and put it on a record turntable. Start the turntable and watch the spiral for one minute. If you then look away and focus on a plain, flat surface, you should still see a spiral, which moves in the opposite direction to the one on the turntable. This effect is probably caused by the tiring of neurons registering movement in the first direction and the subsequently noticeable random firings of nerves which detect movement in the opposite direction.

4 Patterns
For some reason, the brain seems to organize random visual information into patterns – perhaps to aid in the assimilation and categorization of data. The night sky picture, (above left) looks pretty much like any other bit of the sky until we superimpose the artificial image of the Big Dipper (above). Instantly, the random scattering of stars has been mapped and recognized.

©DIAGRAM

Perception: 2

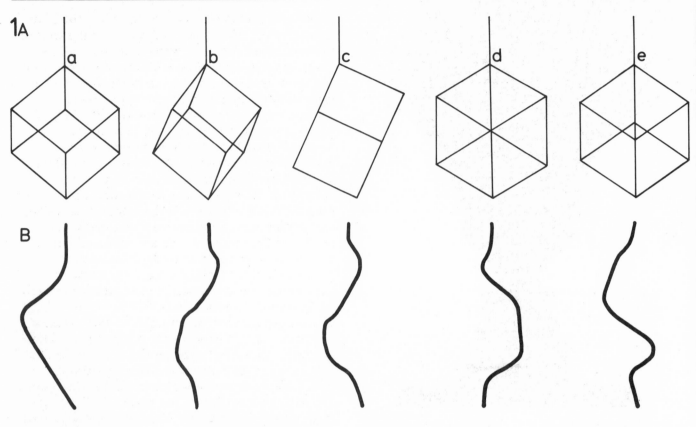

a   b   c   d   e

B

1 Visual Clues
We rely upon being given enough information through our eyes for the brain to interpret correctly the things we see.
A A suspended revolving wire cube eventually gives the brain enough clues to make out its form. Though view **c** is unclear, and **d** and **e** look like hexagons, views **a** and **b** are sufficient to

tell us that it is a box.
B A revolving piece of bent wire never reveals its true form, as there are not enough clues for the brain to comprehend it.

2 Closure
The cards below form part of a memory test, in which the person tested is shown a series of cards, each giving more detail than the last. The aim of the task is to recognize the object at the earliest possible stage, and it is used as a general test of intelligence and alertness. When the test is repeated later on, recognition should take

place at a much earlier stage, as memory fills in the gaps in the drawings.

2

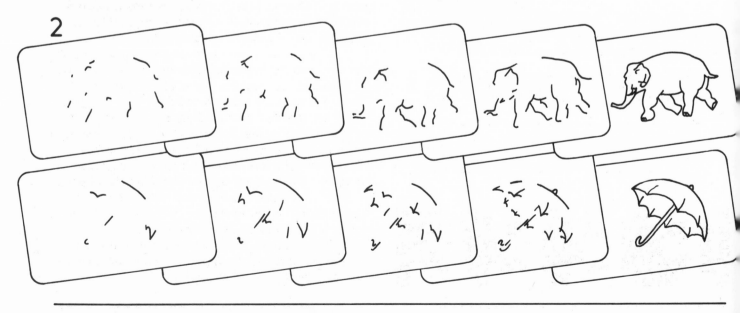

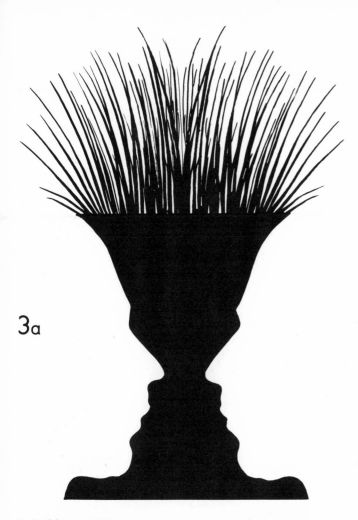

3a

Awareness and Thought

To perceive an object seen by the eyes, the brain takes the signals of light and movement encoded by neurons at the back of the brain and relates them to neurons dealing with memory and often emotion. In this way how we perceive what we do depends at least partly on our experience. Psychologists have shown this with the help of many ingenious experiments. For instance, research reveals that different interests or backgrounds make men and women, primitives and city dwellers, interpret certain pictures differently. Research also shows that, deprived of visual clues that help us judge distance and size, our perception of objects may become wildly faulty. In the same way we are confused when shown an object and its background with the normal tonal contrast reversed, so that what experience tells us should be the figure is in fact the background. Even more confusing is the ambiguous picture: two images in one. Because our minds can attend to only one image at once, our perception shifts back and forth between the two as we try to make both fit an image in our mind. This concept of mental model making may explain closure – the brain's ability to fill in gaps in pictures – for example, the outline of a spotted dog whose silhouette merges with a dappled background.

Evidence that perception indeed involves matching real objects with mental images emerged in a 1980 report by the English neuropsychologist E.T. Rolls. This scientist announced the discovery of three small brain regions connected to the visual cortex – each dealing with a special aspect of perception. In a part of the hypothalamus deep in a monkey's brain, Rolls located neurons that were stimulated by the sight of something edible but nothing else. These neurons emitted impulses when the monkey saw an apple, but a rubber ball left them silent. Near thalamus and hippocampus Rolls found "recognition" neurons. These fired when the monkey saw a familiar object – a big red ball; they ignored a small black ball, an object the monkey had not seen before. Thirdly, in the brain's sensory-motor cortex area Rolls tracked down what we might call "discriminative recognition" neurons. These could tell one familiar object from another. They disregarded red balls or food, but responded to faces – monkey or human; large or small; any color; upright or inverted.

The model-making or hypothesizing that goes on in perception must play a part in that multi-process mental activity we call thought.

3 Ambiguous Pictures
The brain is only capable of perceiving one image at a time in the above picture (a). First we see a vase, then two people about to kiss. But the brain cannot enable us to visualize two people kissing the vase. The two drawings below show how memory may sometimes fail us. The three-pronged figure (b) is impossible to understand as a whole, even though model-making memory helps us to make sense of parts of it. Memory accustoms us to seeing things in certain ways, so we may be confused when the usual order is reversed – what do you see first at the bottom of this page (c), black blobs or a white word?

b

c

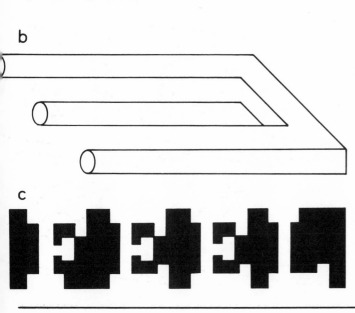

©DIAGRAM

Thought

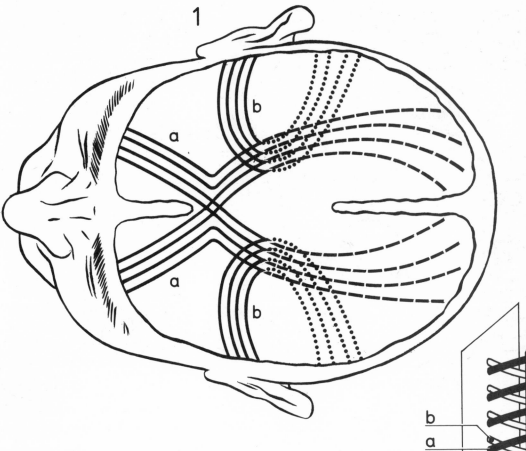

1 Thought as a Hologram
One intriguing theory puts forward the proposition that memory and abstract thought are like a hologram. This theory is based on experimental evidence which shows that memory is not confined to particular areas of the brain but is distributed throughout. Incoming visual (**a**) and auditory (**b**) pathways converge and interfere (left and below), permanently encoding experience as a chemical memory trace on nerve pathways. These memories can be recalled for the purpose of abstract thought and, like a hologram which holds the entire image on every chip of its plate, damage to the brain may not result in loss of remembered experience.

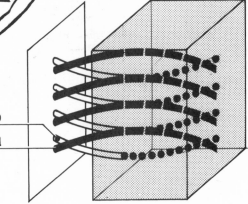

Trying to investigate what goes on in our heads when we think is a problem that has intrigued scientists for centuries.

Psychiatrists and neurologists traditionally denied that science could explain intellect in terms of brain function. Psychologists disagreed, but their bid to explain thought as an association of ideas ignored the fact that thought is so often purposeful. Believing mental activity is just a response to external stimuli, behaviorists discounted the mind, and claimed that "thought" is just forming unspoken words.

Thus experts have not even agreed about what thinking means. For psychologists conducting laboratory tests, thought implies problem solving, but human thought differs from the mechanical processes involved when computers compute. Emotion colors thought. Indeed dreams and schizophrenia hint at two kinds of thought: a rational process involving the cerebral cortex, and "emotional thoughts" going on in the brain's old, inner, limbic system. Perhaps the simplest overall definition of thought is "active uncertainty." Science writer Gordon Rattray Taylor suggested that thinking involves eight stages: (1) recognizing a problem; (2) restraining the impulse to react in a habitual way; (3) investigating what is needed; (4) mentally looking at alternatives; (5) working out a plan; (6) selecting operations to implement it; (7) assessing the results; (8) storing the routine employed for future use.

After half a century of research, thought structure and the seat of reason in the brain remain lively subjects of debate; yet it seems clear that thought involves knowledge, which in turn implies forming and integrating mental concepts at various levels of complexity. The complex, six-layered cortex would seem to possess the organizational capability for this work, though neuroscientist Robert Galambos has suggested that thinking goes on not in the neurons themselves but in the glial cells that support them.

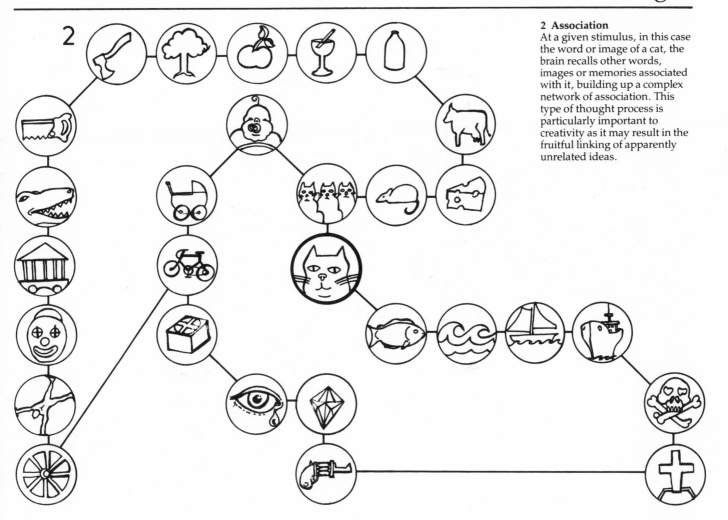

2 Association
At a given stimulus, in this case the word or image of a cat, the brain recalls other words, images or memories associated with it, building up a complex network of association. This type of thought process is particularly important to creativity as it may result in the fruitful linking of apparently unrelated ideas.

Another revolutionary theory, proposed by neurophysiologist Karl Pribram, likens abstract thought to a hologram – a three-dimensional image produced by bombarding a photographic plate with an unfocused pattern of light waves from a split laser beam. One cubic centimeter of plate can handle ten billion bits of information as interference patterns.

Beaming a laser at the plate at the right angle converts these back into the original image. If the brain were organized holographically, this would explain a good deal about its ability to store and process a mass of information.

Pribram's "holographic brain" would encode each memory in a widespread chemical pattern, but Soviet neuropsychologist Alexander Luria, working with brain-damaged patients, points clearly to special parts of the brain controlling different stages of the thought process. For example, people with a damaged occipital – parietal area visualize a simple constructional problem yet lack spatial judgment for solving it. Those with damaged frontal lobes cannot grasp the problem at all.

Scientists have a shrewd idea how the impulses involved in thought reach the brain, and also know by which pathway the impulses leave the brain, but as yet they have little knowledge of how the facts are stored, associated or learned – that is, of the process of thought. It seems most likely that thought involves close, almost simultaneous coordination between many brain regions.

©DIAGRAM

Memory

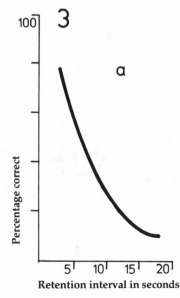

1 Anatomy of Memory
Certain parts of the brain appear to be involved with types of memory. The parietal (**a**), upper temporal (**b**) and occipital (**c**) lobes seem to serve as a short-term memory banks for auditory, visual and kinesthetic (motion perception) impulses.

2 Long-Term Memory
Long-term event memory is stored in the hippocampus (**A**) and in the cortex of the frontal lobes. The cortex of the temporal lobes (**B**) is crucial to abstract memory. The thalami (**C**) are also important to long-term memory.

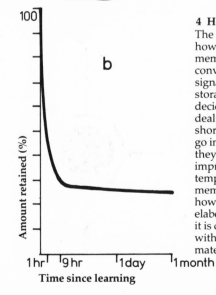

3 Retention of Memory
These two graphs, relating to short-term memory (**a**) and long-term memory (**b**), show the effectiveness of each over an appropriate timescale. Items in the short-term memory are constantly being replaced by incoming items, and so, unless transferred to the long-term memory, they are seldom remembered for more than 20 seconds. Items which have been learned and transferred to long-term memory are also subject to the forgetting process, but the percentage of information retained depends on what kind of information it is – the more organized and meaningful the material, the more will be remembered.

Graph a: Percentage correct vs Retention interval in seconds (5, 10, 15, 20)

Graph b: Amount retained (%) vs Time since learning (1 hr, 9 hr, 1 day, 1 month)

4 How Memory Works
The diagram on the right shows how some scientists think memory works. Our senses convert outside stimuli into signals sent to a temporary storage area where the brain decides how they should be dealt with. Some items go to the short-term memory where they go into a "rehearsal" loop until they are processed. Some impressions go straight from temporary storage to long-term memory. Most information, however, has to go through elaborative processes by which it is categorized and interfiled with previously remembered material.

Human memory can retain an almost unlimited amount of information stretching backward for a lifetime. Our very identity depends upon this record of experience. People have likened memory to a library or computer. New theories about it keep emerging, but studies of individuals with normal and damaged brains, and experiments with animals, convince scientists that memory has several components.

According to one theory, input from the senses to the brain first enters an immediate memory which grasps items for just half a second.

Selected items from the immediate memory pass to the short-term memory. This holds only 5 to 10 items at a time, and for just 10 to 30 seconds. Research shows that the short-term memory stores most information as the coded sounds of words. Auditory, visual and kinesthetic ("motion perception") short-term memory banks seemingly figure in the brain's rear parietal, upper temporal and occipital lobes. New items entering the short-term memory drive out items already there. However, thinking of and mentally repeating items in the short-term memory – a process called rehearsal – shuts out new data and prolongs memory of old.

Items sufficiently rehearsed travel to the long-term memory, designed to span a life's experience. There seem to be three kinds of long-term memory. Stimulus-response memory (the kind involved when a dinner-bell makes a trained dog salivate) employs brain areas below the outer cortex, and survives damage to regions of the brain essential for other kinds of memory. Event memory has limitless capacity for images of past events. Its main centers are the hippocampus and the cortex of the frontal lobes. Abstract memory also has a huge capacity – this time for the meanings of events and objects. Our general store of knowledge, this has its seat in the neocortex, the brain's gray outer layer. Damage to the temporal, parietal or occipital cortex affects abstract memory in different ways.

We can recall items from our long-term memory astonishingly fast thanks to a retrieval system using cues to help us track them down. For example, naming a place where you spent your last vacation may bring back many associated memories. However, memory is not exact. A distorted process called constructive error means that several people will remember the same event quite differently.

Surprisingly, perhaps, forgetting is almost as important as remembering. So-called memory men with total recall have complained because their minds were constantly bombarded by literally unforgettable sensations. One theory explains forgetting as some memories interfering with and blotting out others. Another theory points to the decay of memory traces laid down in the brain. Scientists still seek such memory mechanisms. Most experts see short-term memory as based on an electrical reverberating circuit. Opinions on long-term memory are split. Some think repeated nerve impulses alter junctions, creating new pathways whose activation revives specific memories. Other scientists believe memory-forming involves creating chains of molecules called peptides – maybe one for each new memory created.

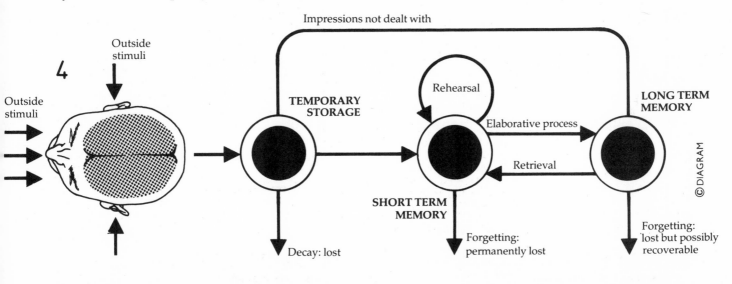

Impressions not dealt with

Outside stimuli

Outside stimuli

Outside stimuli

4

TEMPORARY STORAGE

Rehearsal

Elaborative process

Retrieval

SHORT TERM MEMORY

LONG TERM MEMORY

Decay: lost

Forgetting: permanently lost

Forgetting: lost but possibly recoverable

©DIAGRAM

Language

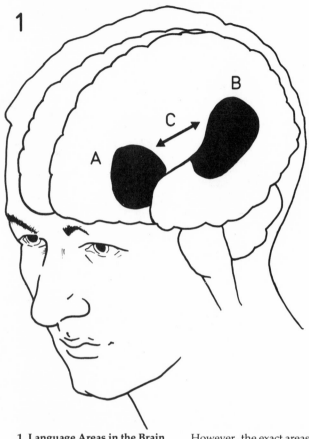

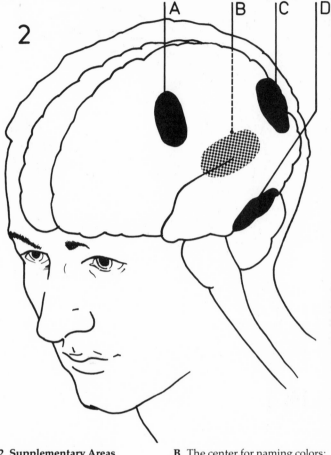

1 Language Areas in the Brain
There are two main areas (above) which have been associated with language:
A Broca's area in the left frontal lobe controls the production of speech.
B Wernicke's area in the left temporal and parietal lobes governs understanding of speech.

However, the exact areas involved vary from person to person. Damage to the links (**C**) between the two main language areas hinders spontaneous speech but leaves repetition unimpaired.

2 Supplementary Areas
Areas governing specific functions associated with language are located (above) in different parts of the brain. The exact locations of these areas vary with individuals; the sites shown here are the most common locations.
A The center for writing.

B The center for naming colors; this is situated at the back of the brain, close to the visual cortex.
C Reading.
D Naming.

More than a century ago scientists began making remarkable discoveries about regions of the brain controlling language. In 1861 the French surgeon Pierre-Paul Broca found local brain damage in the dead patient "Tan-tan," so nicknamed for an affliction that had left him able to utter only these sounds, although understanding what was said to him. After eight more autopsies on similar cases, Broca rightly deduced that the brain's speech mechanism is usually centered in the left frontal lobe – in Broca's area as doctors later christened the bit of the brain involved.

In 1874 the German neurologist Karl Wernicke made another surprising discovery. He found that damage to the left temporal and parietal lobes, farther back in the left cerebral hemisphere, left patients talking grammatical jibberish and unable

to grasp what people said to them. This "language comprehension" region of the cerebrum became known as Wernicke's area.

Subsequent research has shown much more about where language is located. Most information has come from electrically stimulating the exposed cortex of conscious patients and noting where the stimulus temporarily knocks out specific speech or comprehension functions. Thus part of Wernicke's area seems to deal with naming things. Another part permits us to repeat spoken words. Damage to the links between both main language areas hinders spontaneous speech, but leaves repetition unimpaired. Inside the left hemisphere below the visual cortex lies a center enabling us to name colors. Damage to the back of Wernicke's area isolating the rest of it from visual input impairs

3

4

中國

CHINA

3 Damage to Language Areas
Comprehension or production of speech or language may be affected, according to what area of the brain has suffered damage. For example, when there is trauma to the back of Wernicke's area which isolates the rest of it from visual input, the subject may still be able to read a pictographic script like Chinese, but he or she will be unable to read a phonetic script such as English.

4 Mapping Language Areas
When areas of the exposed cortex are electrically stimulated in conscious patients, the functions controlled by those areas may be temporarily disturbed. This can be tested by asking the subject to name objects or repeat words: the sites at which stimulation causes, or fails to cause, error can then be mapped. The diagram (above), showing the induced error sites for three patients, illustrates just how much the language areas vary between individuals.
● Patient 1
■ Patient 2
▲ Patient 3

reading phonetic scripts like English, yet not pictographic scripts such as Chinese. Surprisingly, stimulating brain sites controlling a sequence of mouth movements disrupts not only these but recognition of speech sounds, or phonemes. This underpins a theory that understanding speech involves the brain making an internal "model" for speaking the heard word. Around these sites lie memory regions. Such places occur both in Broca's and Wernicke's areas, suggesting that the old allocation of "speech" and "comprehension" areas is oversimplified.
In fact localization of language areas can differ from person to person, with only the rear third of the frontal lobe – the part controlling motor output of speech – staying constant.
Research into which bits of cerebral cortex control

what aspects of language leaves unexplained how we mentally choose the sounds making up words, and how we arrange these in meaningful order. Behaviorists have explained learning language as a simple conditioning process.
But attempts to teach chimpanzees to speak in the American deaf-and-dumb sign language fail to convince most experts that any creature but man can master the rules of grammar, widely held to be vital to speech. American psycholinguist Noam Chomsky suggests man's brain is born with "deep structures" containing ready-made rules for meaning and grammar. So far they elude detection.

©DIAGRAM

Learning

We have power over other living creatures largely because we outdo them in our ability to use past experience to guide our plans for the future – in other words because we are so good at learning. Thanks to having mastered language we can even add other individuals' experience to ours. Learning affects daily life in dozens of ways – not just our opinions and beliefs, but the way we dress, drive to work, and eat food with a fork. Early this century psychologists experimenting with animals decided that learning depends on the brain associating a stimulus with a response. Russian physiologist Ivan Pavlov discovered that dogs not only salivated at the sight of food – a simple reflex act – they learned to salivate at the sound of a bell rung just before the food appeared. Pavlov called this a conditioned reflex. He argued that conditioned reflexes form a basis for all learned behavior.

Later, psychologists modified Pavlov's ideas. In 1930 the American psychologist Burrhus F. Skinner described operant conditioning. Unlike Pavlov's classical conditioning, which involved persistent change in reflex activity, Skinner's technique caused change in voluntary behavior. Skinner showed that rats accidentally pressing a lever learned to do this deliberately if that act produced food. In other words, he showed that a reward reinforced a response to a stimulus. Skinner's opponents believe that man's great intelligence produces motivations too complex for human learning to be explained just in terms of rewards or punishments.

Whatever the truth, learning certainly produces changes in the brain. We know neurons can change the strength with which they respond to

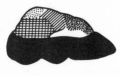
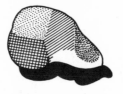

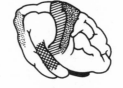

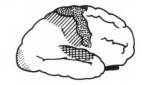

A   B   C   D

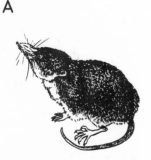
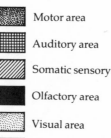
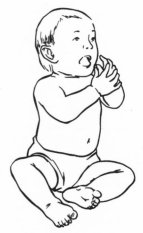

The Uncommitted Brain
The diagram above strikingly shows how man's brain differs from those of lower mammals at birth. Animals which rely strongly on certain senses, for example the ground shrew (**A**) which snuffles for its food, have large areas of cerebral cortex devoted to that sense. The tree shrew (**B**) has the area of visual cortex appropriate to its huge eyes. The brains of the chimpanzee (**C**) and, especially, of man (**D**) are different in that vast areas of cerebral cortex are not committed to sense functions and are thus available for other processes, such as thought and learning.

- Motor area
- Auditory area
- Somatic sensory area
- Olfactory area
- Visual area
- Uncommitted cortex

incoming signals, and so modulate their own transmitted impulses. This readjustment goes on all the time, but especially as we mature, and our ability to learn is at its peak. Maturing also coincides with growing new neuron branches to create a mesh with many possible routes for nervous impulses. Research with octopuses suggests that learning a conditioned reflex strengthens neuron links with small inhibitory neurons in a way that means when one pathway has been used repeatedly, inhibition blocks other routes. Thus the same visual signal eventually triggers an unvarying response.

Exploring the chemistry of learning has also shed light on the general problem. University of California scientists at Berkeley found that rearing rats in a complex, stimulating environment produced marked increases in the brain's weight and protein content, and in activity of enzymes controlling a key neurotransmitter. However, understimulated rats showed no such gains. Research also showed that learning coincides with the brain's manufacture of specific compounds known as peptides (see pp. 102–103).

Whatever happens when we learn, we know that it involves large areas of brain. Thus conditioned reflex learning affects specific areas of positive and negative reward – notably the pleasure and pain centers in the hypothalamus. There is also evidence that learning involves such different regions as the brainstem's reticular formation, that inner emotional brain the limbic system, and of course the corrugated cerebral cortex.

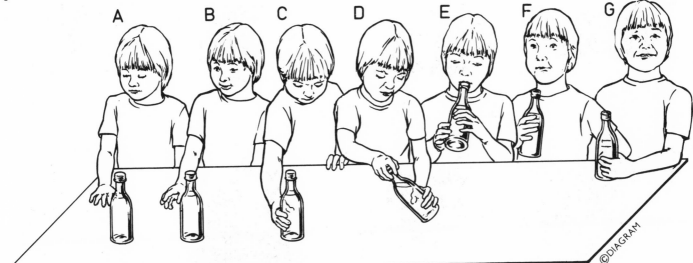

Learning Processes
The sequence of actions (above) demonstrates how many complex learned processes are involved in performing even the simplest of tasks. Well-developed motor skills are essential for the child to be able to reach and grasp the bottle on the table, (**A**), (**B**) and (**C**). Muscular coordination of a high degree is required to unscrew the bottletop (**D**) and raise the bottle to the mouth without spilling what's inside (**E**). According to past experience the child then registers whether the liquid has a good or bad taste (**F**) and thus whether or not it was a good idea to drink it (**G**).

How the Brain Matures
Different areas of the brain grow at varying times and at varying rates, before and after birth. The diagram on the right shows which parts of the cerebral cortex are earliest and latest to mature. Areas which a baby needs first, like centers controlling sensation and movement, are first to mature, but there is great variation within these areas – for example, sensitivity to bright light precedes detailed vision by many months.

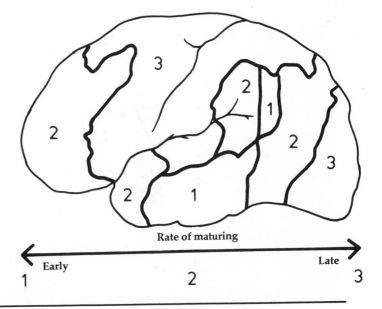

Rate of maturing

Early   Late
1   2   3

Two Brains in One?

Thousands of years ago, Greek thinkers pondering the cleft between the two cerebral hemispheres suggested that we have two brains in one. In fact of course the cleft is not complete, but bridged by the corpus callosum's 300 million nerve fibers. Even so, more than a century ago, studies of brain-damage to one side of the head led English neurologist John Hughlings Jackson to suggest that the left cerebral hemisphere is dominant, for patients with only a functional left hemisphere behaved more like normal individuals than those in which the right half of the brain alone was working. Scientists speculated on the possible effects of dividing a normal brain in two by severing the bridge between both halves. Some argued that the mind would also split in two, others felt it would be indivisible. None guessed such operations would ever happen. They did, though, in the 1950s, as a desperate (and successful) attempt to treat epileptics disabled by frequent and severe attacks of fits.

Roger Sperry and colleagues at the California Institute of Technology were soon learning fascinating facts about the consequences. At first sight, split-brain individuals appeared like ordinary folk: their ability to cycle, sew, play the piano, read or write seemed unimpaired. Yet special tests revealed some strange anomalies. They showed that the left hand of a split-brain person may be doing up one shirt button while the right hand anarchically undoes another. A split-brain person can describe an unseen spoon held in the right hand, but not in the left. Yet he can copy the spatial layouts of drawn solid objects better

1 Major and Minor Hemispheres
In most people the left hemisphere is dominant – as in this diagram. There are many differences between the functions of each side, some of them more subtle than others, but it seems fair to say that in general the major hemisphere deals with analysis, the minor with synthesis.

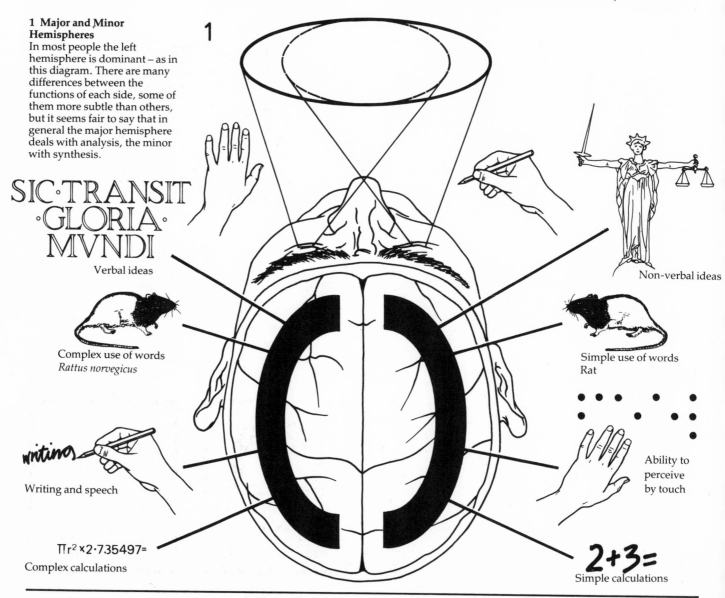

SIC·TRANSIT·GLORIA·MVNDI
Verbal ideas

Non-verbal ideas

Complex use of words
Rattus norvegicus

Simple use of words
Rat

writing
Writing and speech

Ability to perceive by touch

$\pi r^2 \times 2\cdot735497=$
Complex calculations

$2+3=$
Simple calculations

with his left hand than his right, even though right-handed. Because each half of the brain controls the opposite half of the body, tests like these help to show the special functions residing in each cerebral hemisphere.

In most people the left hemisphere is dominant – that is, it speaks, writes, calculates, and thinks logically. But the right or "minor" hemisphere is just as vital in its way. The right hemisphere recognizes faces and shapes, and so helps us to find our way around a town, or get into our clothes. Unlike the logical, analytical left hemisphere, the artistic, musical right one grasps situations as a whole. Thus most intelligence tests explore only the workings of the left half of the brain. Theory has it that left brain hemispheres inspired our Western, strongly verbal, scientific culture, while right brain hemispheres produced the artistic, mystic cultures of the East. Electroencephalograph studies of normal people have helped scientists to work out ratios of left – right dominance. Language dominance lies in the left hemisphere for most adults irrespective of whether right-handed or left-handed. A few people have speech centers in the right hemisphere, a few others in both hemispheres. In young children both hemispheres have speech potential, and speech develops in the right hemisphere if the left is badly damaged. But speech dominance is usually fixed by 10 years of age.

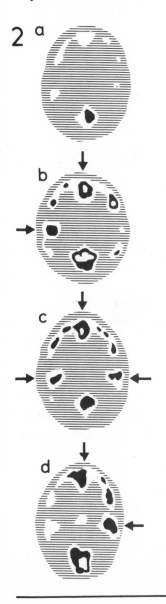

2 Language and Music Centers
Advanced methods of scanning the brain can show us vividly what happens when the brain is engaged in certain tasks. The sequence of scans (left) was taken from a person with left hemisphere dominance. Scan **a** shows the resting brain. Scan **b** was taken while the subject was listening to, and consciously understanding, words. Note how the language area at the side and reasoning area at the front show up darkly. In scan **c** the subject was listening to both words and music – the center in the right hemisphere which recognizes tunes has become active. In scan **d** the subject listened only to music, and the language center on the left has faded.

3 Description and Recognition
One perception test (right) graphically illustrates how the two halves of the brain 'see' things differently. When shown a split picture (**A**) for an instant only, each hemisphere registers a separate image. As the visual pathways cross over within the brain, the left side has 'seen' a man's face, the right a woman's. When the subject is asked to describe the face in the picture, the left side verbally describes a man's face (**B**). But if the subject is shown a set of photographs and asked to point out the face seen, the right side selects the woman's face (**C**) – showing that it is capable of recognition.

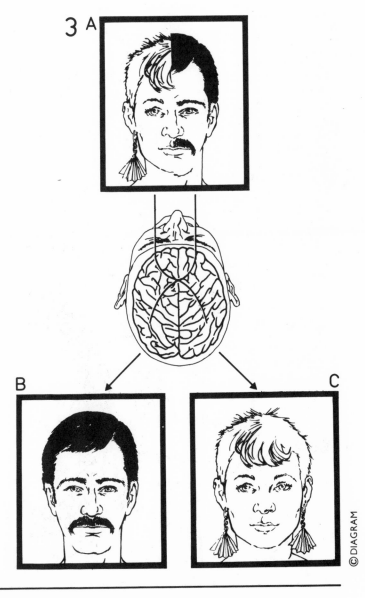

Chapter 7

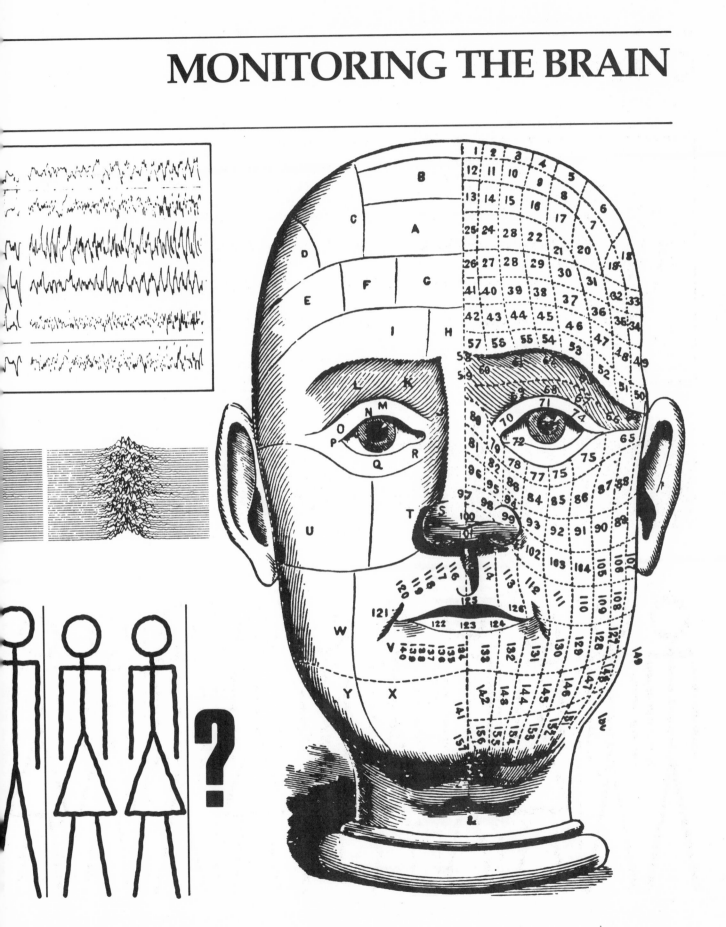

Assessing Intelligence

Assessing intelligence is easier than saying what it is. Various psychologists have come up with entirely different definitions. In 1904, Britain's Charles Spearman claimed intelligence comprised abilities to solve general and specific problems. In 1938 the American Louis Leon Thurstone cited seven primary mental abilities including memorization, reasoning, number and word fluency, perceptual speed, and ability to visualize objects in space. Despite such differences, many psychologists agree that the key ingredient in intelligence is ability to make and use symbols – to construct a mental model of the world outside. This task involves perception, memory and other attributes coordinated in the higher levels of the cerebrum. Each brain hemisphere has some abilities the other lacks. But intelligent activity involves the whole brain and often also receptors in remote parts of the nervous system.

Since the early 1900s, psychologists have developed batteries of intelligence tests for individuals of all ages and every mental level. In each battery, individual tests probe specific mental abilities, for instance language skills involving comprehension, verbal reasoning and vocabulary; and nonverbal skills involving number, arithmetic, and visuospatial ability. To take one example, a revised version of the Stanford-Binet scale for children featured 62 items graded in difficulty for different ages. On this scale, five-year-olds should manage to describe two easy words from a list of 45, copy a square, and repeat a sentence of five monosyllables. Similarly, ten-year-olds should complete the harder tasks expected of their age

1 Intelligence Tests
This intelligence test measures nonverbal performance on the Wechsler Scale. Intelligence tests, however, cannot quantify more complex skills, such as fixing car engines or dealing with children.

2 Distribution Curve
Scores in intelligence tests are standardized so that 100 is the average IQ. 67% of the population have an IQ of between 85–115 – the range of normal intelligence. Fewer than 1% have an IQ of over 150, and the 3% with an IQ of under 70 are considered subnormal.

3 Social Factors
This graph shows the results of three surveys measuring the incidence of mental retardation in children at different ages. Each survey clearly shows an increase at ages 10–14 – the only possible reason for this is the intrusion of social factors, probably increased pressure for high academic performance.

■ First survey
▲ Second survey
● Third survey

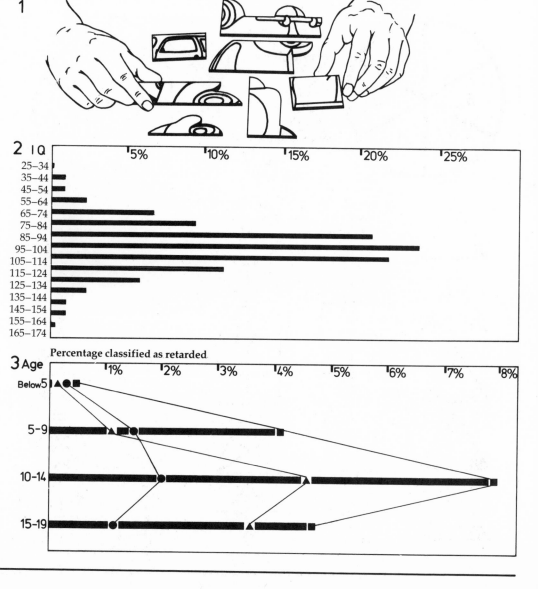

112

group. Tasks actually achieve show mental age. To find an individual's intelligence quotient (IQ) you simply divide mental age by chronological (actual) age, then multiply the answer by 100. For people aged over 15, the Wechsler Adult Intelligence Scale is widely used. This sets two groups of questions: one testing language skills, the other examining nonverbal performance. Standardized scoring of intelligence tests fixes 100 as the average IQ of the population as a whole. More than two-thirds of the population falls within the range 85–115. Fewer than 1 per cent rank above 150 (potential genius level) and the 3 per cent below 70 are ranked subnormal.

Studies of identical twins raised separately suggest that heredity accounts for 80 per cent of an individual's intelligence, environment for only 20 per cent. Yet children in a poor, unstimulating environment score below potential. The wealth gap between blacks and whites in North America may help explain why whites outperform blacks. On the other hand the tests themselves may be to blame: devising questions free of culture bias is notoriously difficult.

IQ tests reveal sexual as well as racial differences: women outperform men when it comes to memory, detail and verbal ability; but men excel in numerical reasoning, mechanical aptitude and gross motor skills.

Despite their uses, IQ tests present a lopsided picture of any individual. They tell us nothing of creativity, initiative, or emotional stability – qualities that can matter even more in life than sheer intelligence.

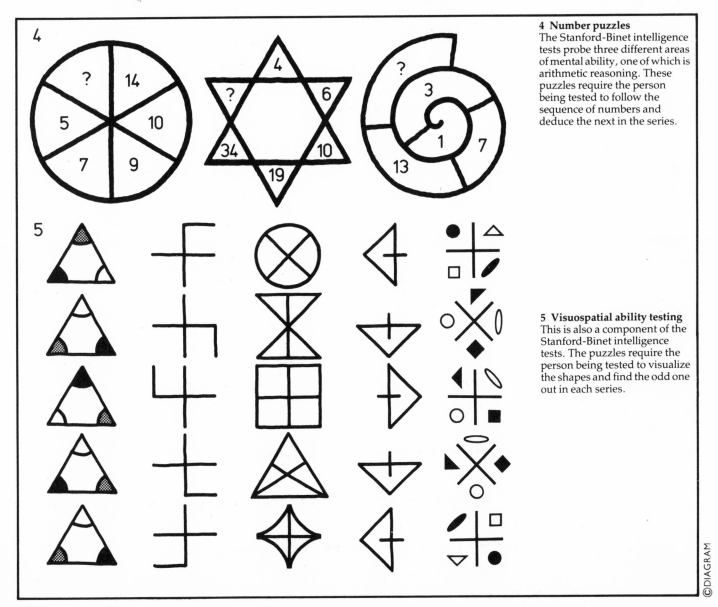

4 Number puzzles
The Stanford-Binet intelligence tests probe three different areas of mental ability, one of which is arithmetic reasoning. These puzzles require the person being tested to follow the sequence of numbers and deduce the next in the series.

5 Visuospatial ability testing
This is also a component of the Stanford-Binet intelligence tests. The puzzles require the person being tested to visualize the shapes and find the odd one out in each series.

©DIAGRAM

Assessing Creativity

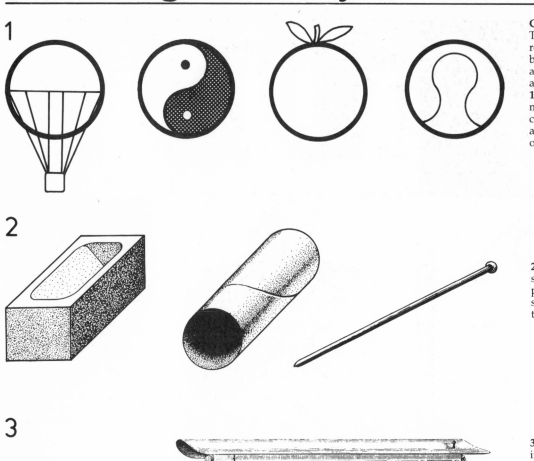

1

Creativity Tests
These tests tend to be less reliable than intelligence tests because the abilities looked for are harder to quantify – there are no right or wrong answers.
1 This test involves drawing as many objects as possible from a circle. Creativity can be assessed from the number and originality of images.

2 A similar type of test involves suggesting as many uses as possible for everyday objects such as a brick, a cardboard tube, and a knitting needle.

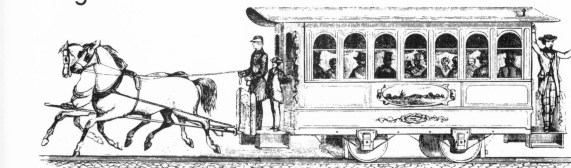

3 A third test involves inventing a story around a given picture. One person might describe this as an early horse-drawn tram, another as a group of nostalgic commuters' answer to the energy crisis.

The last two tests, which require verbal responses, are considered more useful and reliable than the first.

There can be no doubt that some people are better at creating new ideas than others. Artists, poets, composers, philosophers, and pioneering scientists all share a creative spark. Yet measuring creativity is much more difficult than measuring intelligence. This is because intelligence implies ability to solve a problem with a pre-established answer, while creativity's end product is by definition something new.

However, tests developed by psychologists late in the 1950s and early in the 1960s revealed a good deal about the kind of thinking creativity involves. Instead of asking questions with only one correct solution, the psychologists devised open-ended questions affording scope for many answers, each arguably valid.

One such type of question involves suggesting as many uses as possible for some common object, a brick or barrel for example. Another test is drawing as many objects as possible from a circle. Inventing a story around a given picture is a further favorite creativity test, and one producing an astonishing variety of responses. Shown a picture of a man smilingly relaxed inside an airliner, one child described him as a businessman returning home after a successful meeting. To another child he was flying from Reno after divorcing his wife whose slippery face-cream had made her head slide about annoyingly in bed at night. Now the man was thinking happily of the fortune he would make from the nonskid face-cream he had just invented.

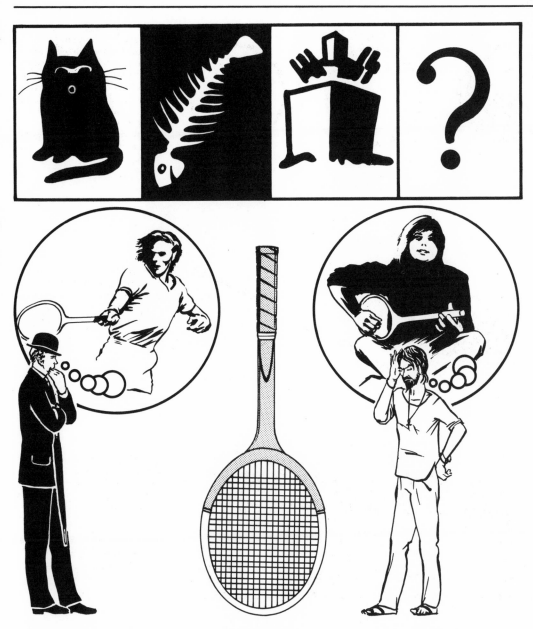

4 Free Association
Creativity may show itself in an ability to relate apparently unrelated objects. The process of free association, in which the mind leaps from one image to another, is therefore a useful test in measuring creativity.

5 Creative Thinking
A convergent thinker, typified by the man on the left, tends to see things in a conventional way and is generally conformist in attitude. However, a divergent thinker, shown on the right, is spontaneously more creative. When shown a common object, the convergent thinker makes a conventional association, whereas the divergent thinker extrapolates from the given image to form a new one.

Psychologists argue that such children represent personalities with two ways of thinking. The first child was a convergent thinker – the type that tends to simplify: approaching problems logically and seeking conventional solutions. The second child was a divergent thinker – the type that seeks new, nonconformist answers; here using the stimulus of given information merely as a base on which to build a complex structure that sprang unprompted from the thinker's mind.
"Divergers" tend to be independent-minded, spontaneous, self-reliant, and rebellious against authority. "Convergers" tend to be less creative, and much more conformist in their attitudes. They tend to score higher than divergers in conventional intelligence tests.

True creativity needs some qualities possessed by both. The creative process involves collecting all facts needed for solving a problem, and logically testing them. But the final answer to a problem often leaps from the subconscious, while an individual is relaxed.
Arguably, creativity – like the hallucinations of a schizophrenic – owes much to the behavior of specific brain cells. Yet creativity implies more than a mind teeming with ideas. There must be judgment and selection, too: the same everyday procedure that the brain employs when we recognize a friend or pick our way through puddles. The creative process can even be laboriously slow: many a great poem has been repeatedly revised.

©DIAGRAM

Testing Brain Functions

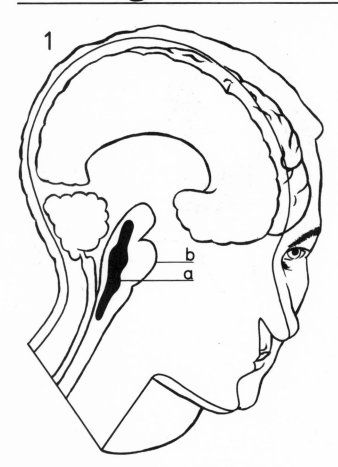

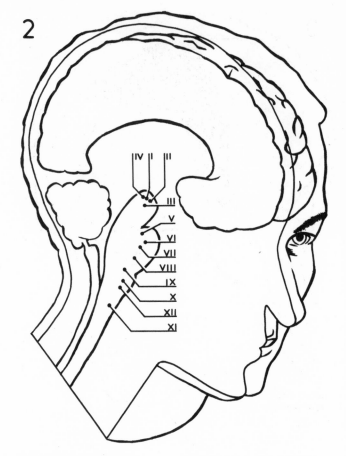

1 Tests for Consciousness
The reticular formation (**a**) in the brainstem (**b**) connects with all major parts of the central nervous system, so tests for consciousness check that this area is still functioning correctly. Responses to light (pupil size), pain (pinching the skin), and noise give an indication of the degree of brain damage.

2 Tests on Cranial Nerves
The sensory input from the twelve cranial nerves, shown above, can be tested by asking the patient to smell through each nostril (olfactory), by visual acuity tests (optic) and by movements of eyelid and eyeball and pupil reflex (oculomotor, trochlear and abducent). Tests for other cranial nerves require the patient to hear, speak, swallow, shrug shoulders, whistle, frown, smile and poke the tongue out straight.

Just as driving a vehicle may reveal defects to a skilled mechanic, so putting the nervous system through its paces helps to tell a doctor how well a patient's brain and related structures work. Simple tests or questions in home or surgery cover mental status, emotional state, and inputs to and outputs from the central nervous system. This history is often very helpful in diagnosis.

If a patient seems unconscious, a doctor tries rousing him by stimuli such as pinching the skin. If the patient can be roused, the doctor tests ability to perceive, react to and recall more stimuli, and ability to think at normal speed.

Psychologists testing intellectual functions find out how well a patient can attend to tasks in hand. They check short-term and long-term memory and rapid recall. They discover how well the patient speaks or writes, and understands spoken and written words; and how well he can calculate, spell, and reverse letters of a word. Doctors test abstract thought by having patients explain proverbs. Other tests of intellectual function cover ability to name and show the use of common objects; use on command of different parts of the body; and awareness of person, time, place. Noticing the patient's emotional condition all through the clinical examination may offer clues to certain forms of mental abnormality.

A separate battery of tests probes the brain's sensory input from the cranial nerves. For instance, holding small bottles of distinctively scented substances to each nostril in turn may show whether the first cranial nerve is fully functional. Visual-acuity and visual-field tests

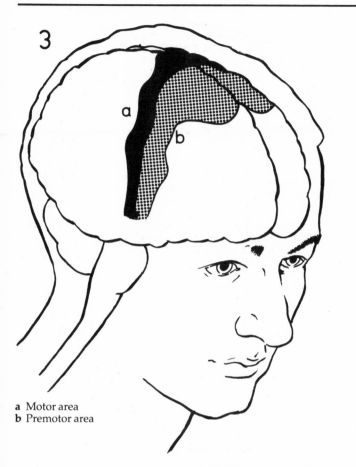

3

a Motor area
b Premotor area

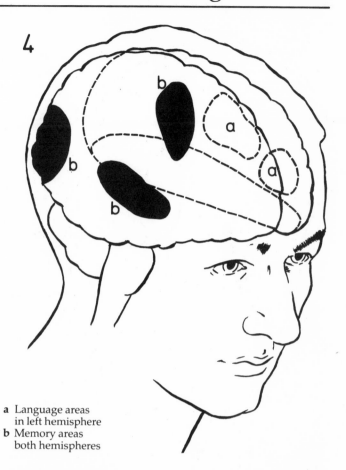

4

a Language areas
   in left hemisphere
b Memory areas
   both hemispheres

3 Motor System Tests
Damage to motor nerve centers in the brain or cerebellum may produce symptoms such as poor balance, lack of muscular coordination and inability to point or to trace a specified shape. Tests therefore include trials of coordination, such as asking the patient to walk heel-toe along a line, or to touch the nose with a forefinger, first with eyes open then with eyes closed. Other tests monitor muscle power, muscle tone and reflexes.

4 Language and Memory Tests
When areas of the brain governing speaking, reading and writing are damaged, these abilities are affected in varying degrees. However, the speech center usually lies in the dominant hemisphere and if this is affected, the other side of the brain may assume its duties. Damage to temporal lobe and hippocampus affects short-term memory. This can be tested by asking the patient to repeat a short sequence of numbers.

indirectly probe the second cranial nerve. Other tests involving eyeball and eyelid movement and pupil reflex between them cover nerves 3, 4 and 6. Light-touch and pinprick sensitivity over the face help to show fifth nerve function. Being able to hear, speak, swallow and shrug shoulders normally; to whistle, frown, smile and poke the tongue out straight helps indicate that the remaining cranial nerves are operational.
Motor system tests evaluate nerve centers or nerves controlling or supplying muscles. Doctors check such things as bodily balance, posture and coordination. They may ask a patient to stand unsupported with eyes closed and feet together, or to walk heel-toe along a line. Coordination tests include touching the tip of the nose with the forefinger tip, eyes open, then eyes closed. A patient lying on a bed may be asked to try to lift one leg to touch the doctor's finger with a toe. Carefully selected tests may show if a coordination problem involves peripheral nerves, or the cerebellum or another region of the brain.
The higher centers of the nervous system are certainly involved in consciously interpreting sensations, for instance numbers traced invisibly upon the skin. Doctors may also have a patient try to recognize common objects by their shape, when handled but not seen.
Coupled with the patient's own account of symptoms suffered, tests like these may reveal specific combinations of defects, pointing to trouble in a specific center in the brain. But more sophisticated tests may be required to show exactly what the trouble is and where it lies.

©DIAGRAM

Mapping the Brain

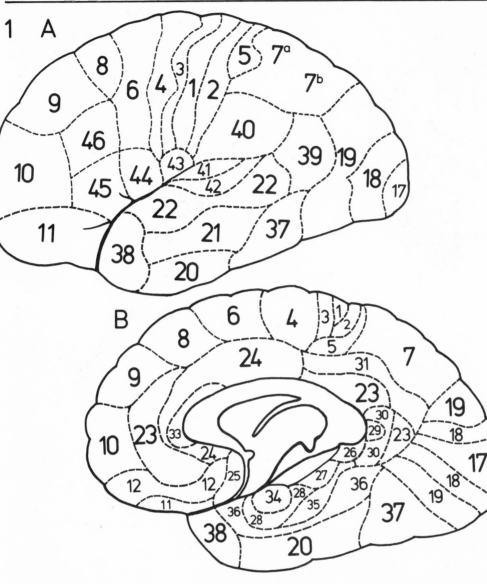

1 A

B

A

B

1 Brodmann's Maps
These maps are chiefly of use as a guide to the different cell structures of the brain, but certain areas have been linked with particular activities – for example, area 17 is associated with sight.
A This map shows numbered areas on the outer surface of the left cerebral hemisphere (for relative position, see top).
B This map shows these areas on the inner side of the right hemisphere (see also above).

Mapping the brain's regions and their functions is an immense and incomplete task. Here we just summarize some of the techniques employed. Special ways of staining brain cells and slicing up the brain enable researchers to divide each cerebral hemisphere into about four dozen numbered areas based on local differences of nerve-cell and fiber structures, and named for Korbinian Brodmann who identified them. Yet the so-called Brodmann areas give no comprehensive guide to where different cerebral functions lodge. Neurologists began locating these as early as the 1860s by noting specific personality or behavior changes caused in epileptic patients suffering damage to local regions of the brain. Electrically monitoring behavior produced in or from those

regions later enabled researchers to map the motor and sensory strips in both cerebral hemispheres. In and after the late 1920s the Canadian neurosurgeon Wilder Penfield probed motor, sensory and so-called psychic areas with 2- and 3-volt currents fired from a single electrode tip touching the exposed brains of conscious patients (less horrific than it sounds, for the brain itself remains insensitive to pain). In fact Penfield's electrodes "froze" the touched areas, but sparked activity in remote but functionally related brain regions connected to them.
Stimulating electrodes implanted deep inside the brain has also shown connections between certain hidden structures and emotions.
Trickier than recording artificially stimulated brain

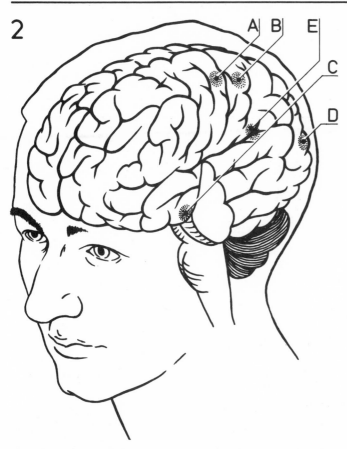

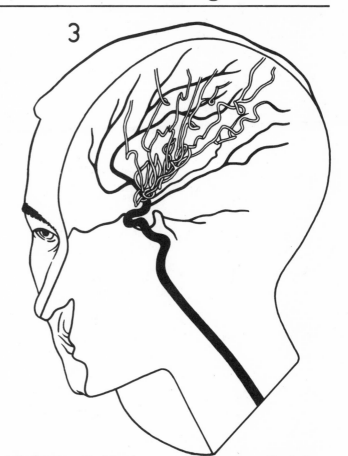

2 Stimulation of Brain Sites
Probing the brain with electrodes helps to establish which areas are associated with particular physical sensations, or sensations affecting the consciousness. The diagram shows the left cerebral hemisphere. Stimulation in the somatic motor cortex (**A**) and the sensory motor cortex (**B**) produce movement and sensation respectively in the right hand. Stimulation in the speech cortex (**C**) produces aphasia; in the visual-sensory cortex (**D**) it produces a sensation of light. Stimulation in the interpretative cortex in the fissure of Silvius (**E**) activates a stream of consciousness.

3 Radioisotope Tracking
Advancements in radioisotope science in recent years have enabled neurologists to produce accurate "maps" of an individual's brain. Radioactive tracers may be introduced into the cerebrospinal fluid, or into the circulatory system (above). As the chemical moves through the arteries of the brain, its path can be tracked with scanners sensitive to the tiny amounts of radiation emitted; abnormalities in the path can be noted on the scanner's visual readouts, and may be helpful in diagnosing neurological problems.

activity is monitoring the natural working of individual brain cells. Yet this, too, has been accomplished, by having a microelectrode touch or penetrate a cell, amplifying the electrical pulses given off and viewing these on an oscilloscope. This is how we know that different cells in the visual cortex respond to individual angles, or movements in particular directions.

Thanks to PETT (see page 123) scientists can also study groups of cells at work, even identifying combined sensory-motor brain areas by relating changes in their glucose uptake to specific mental and physical activities.

PETT relies on tagging groups of cells with radioactive substances, and then observing their behavior. But PETT is only one way of tracing the pathways in the brain – trails that laid end to end would reach at least to the Moon and back. There are also ways of tagging cells selectively to find which nerve connects to which.

These techniques include injecting brains with fluorescent dyes or amino-acid molecules including radioactive isotopes of certain atoms, then tracing their passage through the brain. Another promising technique is developing antibodies (natural defenses of the body) that lock onto specific types of nerve cell. This offers hope for mapping nerve systems according to their roles.

Only when scientists have mapped millions of connections may we truly comprehend the immensely versatile computers in our skulls.

©DIAGRAM

Studying Brain Waves

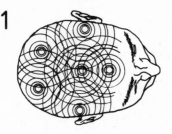

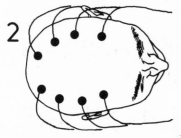

Detecting Brain Waves
1 Electric signals ripple across the brain as millions of brain cells fire repeatedly.
2 Electrodes at intervals along the head reveal a set of brain-wave traces.
3 One wave trace may combine waves of several frequencies (here shown below it).

4 Measuring Brain Waves
Brain waves are measured in cycles per second.
a Cycle: one complete oscillation.
b Frequency: oscillations per second; the more there are the higher the frequency.
c Amplitude: half the height from peak to trough in a single oscillation.

Electroencephalography (literally "electric-in-head-writing") is a method of gleaning clues to the state of the brain by detecting its output of minute electrical "ripples." Their immediate cause is changes in electrical charges on different parts of the brain, due to synchronized activity by large groups of neurons. Some brain waves reflect events deep down in the brain; others are evidently influenced by eye movements. Each individual's brain-wave activity is as unique and distinctive as his or her fingerprints.

Electroencephalogram (EEG) readings involve attaching a person to an electroencephalograph, a device with wires, an amplifier, electromagnetic pens, and paper revolving on a drum. One end of each wire is "glued" to the subject's scalp. Eight or even more wires may be affixed at carefully measured intervals. The wires' other ends are attached to the amplifier. This takes the brain's electrical impulses of 100 microvolts (one ten-thousandth of one volt) or less and magnifies them one millionfold. Traced on paper by pens, these impulses appear as rows of oscillating waves. Brain waves vary in frequency and amplitude, but it is usually frequency that tells us most about what is going on in the brain. In normal individuals frequency varies with alertness or activity, but some types of wave occur more in certain parts of the brain than in others.

Scientists group brain waves into four main types according to the frequency. From high to low frequency these types are know as beta, alpha, theta and delta waves. Beta and alpha rhythms are the commonest in healthy, wakeful adults. Slower rhythms persist in sleep, early childhood and serious illness. Epileptic seizure reveals sudden fluctuation in amplitude. In localized brain malfunction abnormal waves tend to flow only from the part of the brain that is affected.

Computerized electroencephalography assists the detection of evoked potentials – minute voltage changes induced in the brain as it responds to specific sights or sounds. This process – which selects insignificant signals from the general background of electrical activity – shows that attention, expectancy and making instant decisions involve different brain waves. Evoked potentials techniques also aid the study of brain conditions in the newborn, in some children with learning problems, in the comatose, and in victims of stroke, brain tumor and multiple sclerosis.

For studying certain brain conditions, brain-scan devices have largely outmoded EEG techniques.

5 Types of Wave

The four types of brain wave are named for Greek letters. ·

δ Delta waves (1–3 cycles per second): due to brain tumors. Also found in sleep and in early infancy.

θ Theta waves (4–7 cycles per second): dominant at ages 2–5 and in psychopaths, or evoked by frustration.

α Alpha waves (8–13 cycles per second): prominent in adults with eyes closed and the mind at rest. Best obtained from the back of the head.

β Beta waves (faster than 13 cycles per second): mainly seen in adults, and best found in the middle and front of the head – related to the brain's sensory-motor areas.

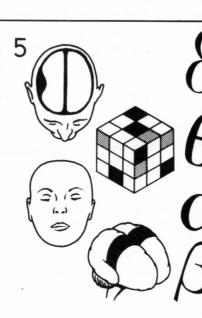

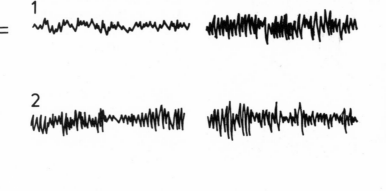

Eyes open

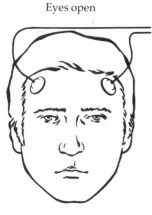

Eyes shut

1

2

3

Alpha Wave Types

A research team working in England in the 1940s discovered that alpha rhythms held clues to certain aspects of human personality. The team identified three main types of people according to their alpha wave activity.

1 Type R, for "responsive." In these adults alpha rhythms predominate when the eyes are shut and the mind is relaxed. The rhythms are only lost or "blocked" on opening the eyes or making mental effort. About two-thirds of all tested people were type R. Such people can form mental images to help them think but do not habitually do so.

2 Type P for "persistent." Alpha rhythms persist in these individuals even when they open their eyes and grapple with mental problems. About one-sixth of all adults seem to fit into this category. Type P people perceive by sound or touch much better than by forming visual images.

3 Type M, for "minus." These people show no noticeable alpha rhythms whether eyes are shut or open and minds blank or busy. About one-sixth of all adults are type M, and always think in visual images.

Grey Walter, who led this research, suggested a simple test to help anyone discover his or her own alpha type. Walter's test goes like this. Shut your eyes. Imagine a big painted cube. Imagine you cut it in half across one side. Cut each half in half again. Cut them once more at right angles. Try to picture the tiny cubes you have made. How many of their sides are unpainted? Did you have to work out the answer or did you seem to see the cubes? If so, did you see their color? Anything else? If you saw no picture you may be a P type. If you saw more than the fewest necessary details you may be an M type. If you saw an image that was just enough to let you answer you are probably type R. P's find visual problems difficult. Abstract problems puzzle M's. R's tend to be the most versatile of problem solvers.

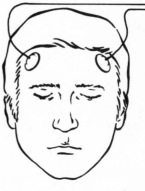

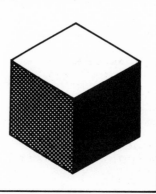

©DIAGRAM

Scanning the Brain

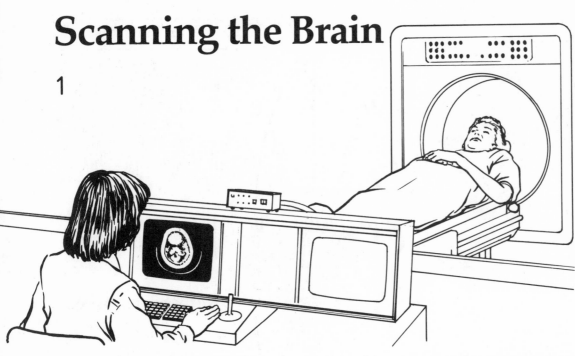

1 Scanning the Brain
Some early techniques for diagnosing disorders of the brain had the disadvantage that they involved invading the brain or its surroundings, a potentially risky procedure. New diagnostic methods, such as CAT (shown left) and PETT, are much safer and are capable of giving us a much clearer picture of the brain's anatomy and how it works in sickness and in health. These sophisticated techniques, combining relatively low-dose radioactivity and the ingenuity of computers, enable a diagnosis to be made quickly, without requiring a long stay in hospital.

Functional tests and electroencephalography indicate the brain's condition only indirectly. Increasingly subtle diagnostic aids now let doctors probe the actual contents of the brain.
Well-tried techniques include spinal tap (lumbar puncture) – inserting a hypodermic needle in the spinal canal of the lower spine. Spinal taps can reveal pressure in the central nervous system, and withdrawing cerebrospinal fluid aids diagnosis of infection and some other conditions. Air injected via the spinal canal fills the cavities, or ventricles, inside the brain. X-rays of the air-filled ventricles, called pneumoencephalograms, may reveal brain atrophy or tumors. Myelograms are X-rays where radio-opaque substances injected in the spinal canal help to show up slipped disks, tumors and spinal injuries. Variations on such techniques include the ventriculogram and arteriogram. In the first, a doctor injects air into the ventricles directly through the brain. In the second, a radio-opaque substance injected in an artery helps to reveal the condition of the blood vessels that supply the brain.
There are snags with these techniques, however. All involve invading the brain or its immediate surroundings, some riskily. Also, certain tests require a stay in hospital, and none of those described gives a detailed image of the brain.
By the 1970s, though, new, noninvasive ways of peering at the brain were revolutionizing diagnosis.
Echoencephalograms using ultrasound reflections bounced back from the brain surface betray intracranial abnormality and midline structures. But the most dramatic developments include computer-aided X-rays showing sections through the brain or scanning its chemical activity.
In computerized axial tomography (CAT), an X-ray tube rotates around a patient's head, bombarding it with narrow X-ray beams. Emerging modified by local variations in brain-tissue density, the beams strike detectors that convert them to electronic signals fed to a computer. This analyzes changes to the X-rays as they traveled through the head, and shows them as a tomogram – a brain cross-section projected on a television screen. CAT scans help doctors pinpoint blood clots, tumors, birth defects and other damage.
An even more sophisticated system is the DSR (dynamic spatial reconstructor). While CAT shows slices of the brain, the DSR reveals it three-dimensionally, and pulsing with activity. Each firing 60 times per second, the DSR's 28 revolving X-ray guns produce 75,000 images in just five seconds – far more than CAT can cope with.
Unlike CAT and DSR, PETT (positron-emission transaxial tomography) bombards detectors encircling the head with radiation emitted from the brain itself. The gamma rays result from radioactive isotopes injected or inhaled by patients as a gas. PETT produces brain maps that vividly reveal how injury or illness alter local blood flow or metabolic activity.
Nuclear magnetic resonance (NMR) – yet another type of brainscan – employs electromagnetic radiation to activate protons in body tissue and build an image of the brain. This safe, painless method shows the clearest pictures yet and promises new certainties in diagnosis.

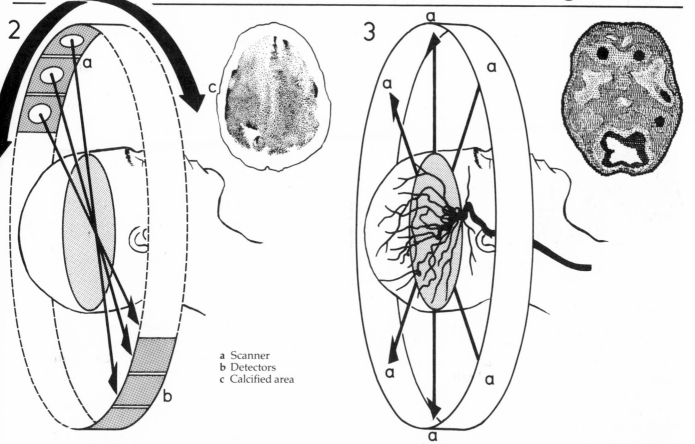

a Scanner
b Detectors
c Calcified area

2 Computerized Axial Tomography (CAT)

The CAT scanner works by sending thin X-ray beams at one degree intervals over 180° in an arc over the patient's head. Lining the 180° arc beneath the head are detectors which measure how the X-ray beams have been modified by variations in tissue density within the brain. Information from the detectors is fed into a computer which builds up an image on a TV screen showing a cross-section of the brain (tomogram). The CAT scan above is of the brain of an epileptic woman and shows a calcified area in the left occipital region which was scarcely visible on ordinary X-rays.

3 Positron-Emission Transaxial Tomography (PETT)

PETT has exciting possibilities because it can show which areas of the brain are active at a particular time and in response to a particular stimulus. Radioactive particles in the brain's blood supply are monitored by detectors (a) around the patient's head.

Active areas of the brain attract most radioactive particles and so show up strongly. The PETT scan above shows intense activity in the visual interpretation region of the brain as the subject looks at a street scene.

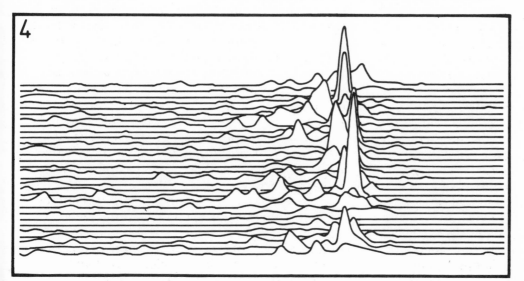

4 Compressed Spectral Array

CSA uses frequency analysis techniques (performed by a computer) to translate EEG information into an easily interpreted pictorial form: a 30- 40 minute clinical EEG recording can easily be presented on a single page. The frequency is plotted along the horizontal axis and each line of the display is generated from 4 seconds of EEG data. The example, (left) is a reading of the alpha-wave rhythm of a normal adult.

©DIAGRAM

Chapter 8

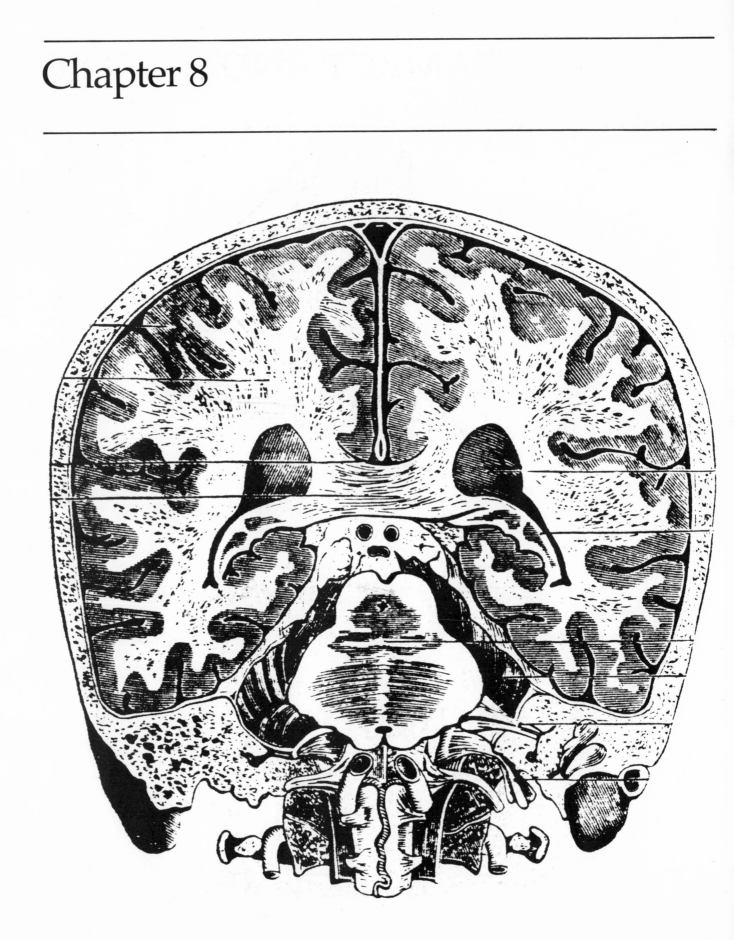

DAMAGE AND DISEASE

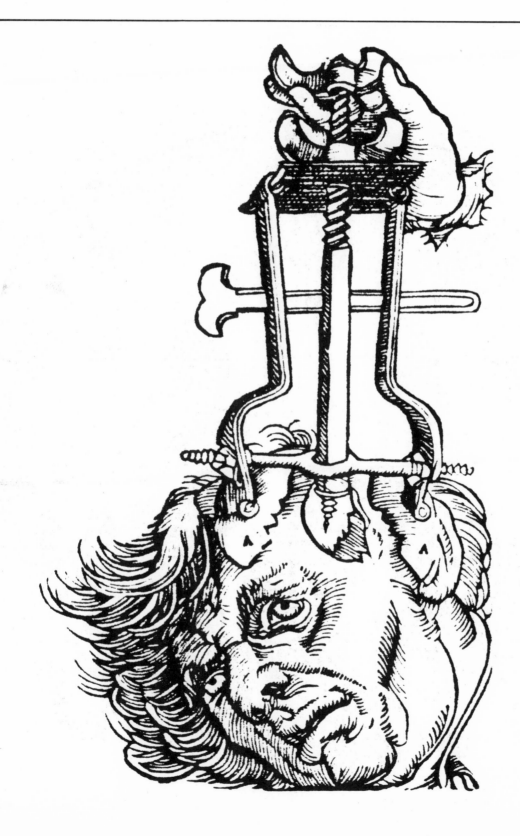

Effects of Brain Damage

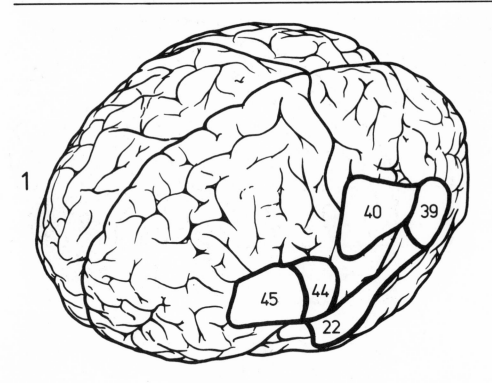

1

1 External Damage
Damage to the outside of the cerebral hemisphere can have various results depending on which area is affected. The diagram shows some areas that are located on the left hemisphere in most people, and which are associated with a specific function or skill.
Areas 44 and 45 are the motor speech areas of Broca. Damage results in an inability to produce connected speech sounds.
Area 22 is associated with recognition of sounds. Damage results in an inability to recognize familiar sounds or to interpret and understand speech.
Area 39 is the visual equivalent of area 22. Failure to recognize objects or understand written language results if this area receives injury.
Area 40 is concerned with interpretation. Injury can result in a failure to interpret the nature of an object by touch, or the loss of awareness of bodily parts and spatial relationships.

Damage, disease or maldevelopment interfering with a specific region of the brain may impair the function that that part controls or helps to coordinate. Here we show some examples of local damage and its effects on senses, bodily control, personality and intellect.

Damage to specific association areas – areas making up most of the cerebral cortex – produces strange phenomena collectively called agnosias, aphasias and apraxias.

People with agnosia fail to notice or recognize certain kinds of familiar things around them. If damage involves the dominant hemisphere's area number 40 (as plotted by brain cartographer Korbinian Brodmann) there will be astereognosis – inability to recognize by touch familiar objects like a coin or ball. Damage to area 22 on the same side of the brain produces auditory agnosia – failure to recognize familiar sounds including spoken words. If area 39 on the same side of the brain malfunctions, a person cannot recognize familiar objects that he sees.

Aphasias are language disorders produced by damage to certain other regions of the dominant hemisphere. Injury to areas 22 and 39 produces sensory aphasia – inability to understand spoken or written words, though these are recognized. If someone cannot use a part of the back of the temperoparietal region he suffers motor aphasia – and cannot meaningfully express his thoughts in speech or writing.

Individuals with apraxias have intact nerve pathways between brain and muscles, yet cannot purposefully carry out skilled, complicated movements. Apraxias include agraphia, inability to write or draw; oral dysphasia, inability to speak articulately; and transmissive apraxia, inability to wash face, brush teeth, comb hair, or perform a similar sequence of tasks to order, while remaining able to complete these acts unthinkingly. Brain regions involved include areas 44 and 45 (oral aphasia), area 40 alias the supramarginal gyrus (transmissive aphasia), other cortex regions, and connecting fibers.

Hippocampus damage may interfere with memory. Prefrontal lobe damage can cause personality disorders.

Deep inside the brain, lesions cause other problems. Thus damage at different points along the visual pathways produces various visual field defects. Failure of the hypothalamus to form the antidiuretic vasopressin (ADH) can cause diabetes insipidus. Certain forms of damage to the thalamus make someone supersensitive to heat, cold, pain and pressure.

2 Internal Damage
The structures inside the brain are extremely complex, so the effects of damage to a particular structure vary considerably depending on exactly which parts have suffered.
A Optic nerve damage leads to partial or total blindness.
B Hypothalamus damage can result in a wide range of effects, from inability to regulate appetite and body temperature, to hormonal and emotional disturbances.
C Hippocampus malfunction interferes with short-term memory.
D Brainstem damage also results in many different defects including loss of pain and temperature sensation if the medulla (**a**) is affected, and weakness or paralysis of muscles if the pons (**b**) or medulla suffer.
E Thalamus malfunction interferes with the transmission of sensations, often resulting in excess sensitivity to pain, heat, and other stimuli.

F The cerebellum is important in balance and fine control of movement. The more obvious effects of damage are lack of equilibrium resulting in a staggering gait and a tendency to fall over, and reduced muscular coordination shown by tremor, slurred speech and disjointed movements.

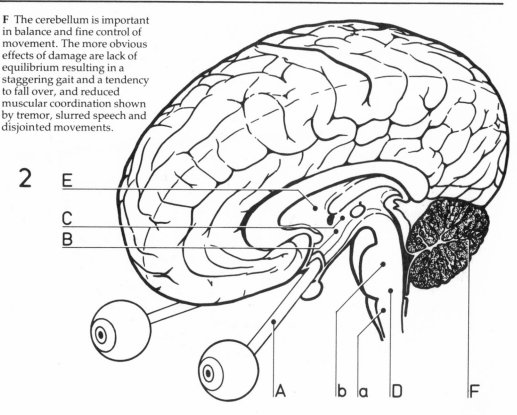

Because nerve tracts from brain to spinal cord cross over in the brainstem, damage to one cerebral hemisphere may paralyze the other side of the body. However, damage to one side of the cerebellum affects body movements on that side. Cerebellar lesions may cause the puppetlike jerky movements of asynergia and dysmetria ("past pointing" – pointing to one side of an object and overshooting); intention tremor; ataxia (walking with a broad-based, "drunken" gait); and dysarthria (speaking in a slurred, staccato fashion). Damage to both cerebellar hemispheres most affects the hands; damage to the middle of the cerebellum so afflicts the trunk that walking and even sitting upright may become impossible. Brainstem damage has different effects depending on which section (midbrain, pons or medulla) is affected, and which segment at that level is involved. For example, one-sided damage to part of the midbrain roof may produce so-called intention tremor and unsteady, broad-based gait. Damage to the basal and medial region of the pons produces double vision and partial paralysis of both sides of the body. Damage to one side of the medulla may make swallowing difficult, banish gag reflex on the same side, and remove pain and temperature sensation from the same side of the

face, the opposite side of the body, and the back of the head. In each case, of course, damage done depends on the nerve pathways involved.
In mentally retarded individuals, brain damage often seems widespread. Examining a brain after death may show that the whole organ has shrunk or never fully grown. Sometimes the glial ("glue") cells of the white matter have spread at the expense of the neurons in the gray matter. Sometimes the white matter itself seems wasted. But there can be local trouble, too, as in the maldevelopment of the cerebellum or the frontal lobes, or local hemorrhage, injury, or infection.
So far researchers have failed to find lesions in the brain to explain such lesser mental problems as dyslexia, or reading difficulty, a disability also affecting spelling. Dyscalculia, calculating difficulty, is another well-known learning problem. About 15 per cent of American school-age children reportedly suffer some learning difficulty or another. Many find that special tuition techniques prove helpful.
The next pages explore specific types of injury and ailment that afflict the brain and what medicine does to minimize their ill-effects.

© DIAGRAM

Problems Present from Birth

1 Congenital Disorders
These include cerebral palsy, hydrocephalus and Down's syndrome (see below). Phenylketonuria and galactosemia are metabolic diseases which may result in brain damage. In most of these a newborn baby shows no external signs of abnormality. Cerebral palsy arises as a result of insufficient oxygen or glucose reaching the brain during birth. Babies with this either move stiffly and with difficulty or exhibit unnatural body movements. Hearing is often impaired.
Hydrocephalus is the excess accumulation of cerebrospinal fluid in the brain. Babies born with this tend to have a larger than normal head. Phenylketonuria and galactosemia are genetically determined abnormalities of the metabolism that result in mental retardation. Until the baby is old enough for this to become apparent, there are no obvious external signs and for this reason it is important that babies undergo biochemical tests soon after birth.

2 Down's Syndrome
Down's syndrome (mongolism) is the result of one chromosome too many. Sufferers typically grow up mentally retarded and frequently have defects of the heart and lungs. However, they are usually affectionate and cheerful children with a fondness for music and dance. Down's syndrome may be recognizable at birth – compare the picture (right) with the top picture of a normal baby.

a Eyes noticeably slanted and close together.
b Ears small and often misshapen.
c Nose often pug-shaped, leading to snuffly breathing.
d Tongue large and often protruding.
e Hands broad and stumpy with only a single crease ("simian line") across the palm.
f Little finger is incurved and often only has two bones and a single crease.
g Feet broad and short with a longitudinal furrow and a wide gap between the first and second toes.

3 Occurrence of Defects
The diagram shows the number of occurrences of babies born with congenital disorders.
A Down's syndrome. 3.5 out of every 10,000 babies born have this defect. If the mother is over 40, the rate rises to 200 (1 in 50 babies).
B Anencephaly. 6 in every 10,000 babies are born with this fatal abnormality in which the brain and top part of the skull are absent. It is more common if the mother is very young or very old.
C Spina bifida. This, often together with hydrocephalus, occurs in 10 out of 10,000 live births.
D Mental subnormality. Excluding those with Down's syndrome, 17 out of every 10,000 babies are born with some degree of mental defect.

Surprisingly many children are born with brain impairment affecting one or more senses, muscle control, mental ability or all three. While some suffer grave mental or physical handicap, others appear almost normal. The root of such a problem may be an inherited defect, damage sustained in the womb, or injury occurring at or after birth. The commonest malformations affecting the brain and spinal cord are hydrocephalus and spina bifida. In hydrocephalus ("water-filled brain") prebirth brain malformation or inflammation traps cerebrospinal fluid in the brain's natural cavities. After birth, fluid dammed up in the head enlarges the skull, and presses hard on the brain, perhaps destroying tissue. The baby suffers fits, blindness, paralysis and death within two years unless fitted with a special tube to drain excess fluid from the brain. Hydrocephalus often occurs with spina bifida ("cleft spine"), a condition where failure of some vertebrae to fuse lets part of the spinal cord protrude.

Brain defects arising before, during or soon after birth account for the many forms of so-called cerebral palsy. Causes include too little oxygen or glucose reaching the brain, or actual injury during a difficult birth. Often damage affects mainly one cerebral hemisphere to produce hemiplegia – weakness or paralysis of the opposite side of the body. Athetosis (involuntary writhing movements of limbs and face) combined with speech difficulty may make someone with cerebral palsy seem mentally strange. Yet many with this condition have normal intelligence. Care during pregnancy and medical skill at the birth may help to prevent babies being born with cerebral palsy.

Several inborn conditions cause serious effects including mental retardation. Of those due to a chromosome disorder the commonest is Down's syndrome (mongolism) which afflicts one baby in every 600 and 2 or 3 per cent of all babies born to mothers aged 40 or more. Caused by an extra chromosome, mongolism produces visible abnormality and stunts mental development. IQ ranges from 33 to 70 (average IQ is 100) and mongol children cannot think in symbols as ordinary people do.

Two important inherited conditions impair the brain by interfering with metabolism. Each involves lack of an enzyme needed to help the body use a compound found in certain foods. About one per cent of mentally retarded people suffer from phenylketonuria. Lacking the enzyme phenylalanine hydroxylase, they cannot use the amino acid phenylalanine in ordinary protein. Accordingly this substance builds up in the blood, damaging the brain. Similarly, sufferers from galactosemia cannot digest galactose, a sugar found in milk. Luckily most babies with these two conditions are spared mental disability if given diets that exclude the substances their bodies cannot metabolize.

Doctors can often predict the chances of having a badly brain-damaged baby. Some women at risk avoid pregnancy or have abortions rather than give birth to individuals forever needing care.

In fact only a quarter of those born mentally retarded need lifelong care. Given sufficient help and stimulation, the rest can learn self-care and useful tasks, performed in sheltered workshops.

4

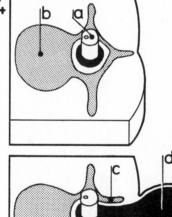

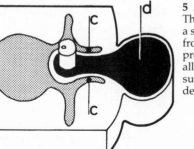

4 Spina bifida
In a fully developed spine (left, above) the spinal cord (**a**) is completely enclosed by the vertebrae (**b**). But in spina bifida (below) one or more vertebrae are open at the back (**c**), allowing spinal fluid (**d**) to pass through and form a bulging sac along the spine.

5 Amniocentesis
This technique involves drawing a sample of the amniotic fluid from the uterus during pregnancy. Amniocentesis allows some fetal abnormalities, such as spina bifida, to be detected before birth.

5

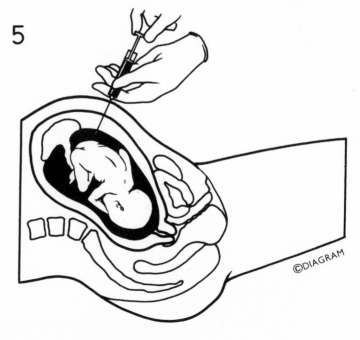

©DIAGRAM

Infection

Infection and inflammation can attack the brain or other parts of the central nervous system, sometimes with serious results. Luckily, the body's defenses make such events fairly uncommon.

Infective agents include bacteria, fungi and viruses. Sometimes one involves the whole nervous system, but certain germs specialize in attacking special regions. Infections involving a particular part of the nervous system are named accordingly. Of the two major types found in the head, encephalitis ("brain inflammation") affects the brain, meningitis afflicts the meninges – the brain's protective outer coverings.

1

1 Sources of Infection
Bacteria, viruses and fungi can enter the brain via several routes.
a Direct penetration through a wound in the skull.
b Spread of bacteria from an abscess in an infected ear.
c Spread of infection from the nasal sinuses after a cold, influenza, etc.
d Infection may be carried by the blood stream from a distant part of the body.
e Viruses such as that causing rabies travel through a peripheral nerve toward the brain. The time the virus takes to reach the brain depends on the distance of an infected bite from the head – rabies may take many months to develop after a bite in the leg.

Organisms sometimes invade the brain directly through a wound penetrating the skull, or from an infected ear or nasal sinus. Some organisms reach the brain from other parts of the body via the bloodstream or by tracking through nerves.
The nature of any disease in the nervous system depends on the organism involved, how fast the infection develops, and where it is located.
Infections inside the head tend to produce inflammation with nausea, vomiting and fever. Light may hurt the eyes, and the patient may feel drowsy, fall unconscious or suffer confusion, convulsions and partial paralysis. Meningitis may produce a stiff neck. Fear of water (hydrophobia) and maniacal behavior can be features of rabies (its name is Latin for "madness").
Brain infections may visibly affect the brain. In meningitis pus and inflamed blood vessels may block the flow of cerebrospinal fluid between the brain's innermost meningeal coverings, and fluid presses on the brain. Encephalitis inflames cells in the cerebral cortex, white matter, basal ganglia and brainstem, actually killing off numbers of neurons.
Rabies – a viral disease spread by saliva from the bite of an infected creature or person – leaves traces called inclusion bodies in the brain's cerebellum, hippocampus and medulla. Poliomyelitis – caught by breathing in a virus – attacks motor neurons in the spinal cord and sometimes the brainstem, to cause paralysis and muscle wasting.
Treatment depends on the cause of the disease. Antibiotics help to cure meningitis due to bacteria. Unfortunately nothing kills the encephalitis virus, and doctors can only give drugs to lower the patient's temperature, control convulsions, and, if needs be, draw off spinal fluid to reduce fluid pressure on the brain. However, encephalitis-like symptoms sometimes spring from an abscess due to local brain infection that can be treated by antibiotics and drawing pus from the abscess through a hypodermic needle.
These infections vary in their outcome. Rabies is almost always fatal once symptoms appear. Meningitis can often be completely cured, encephalitis may lead to total recovery or death. Either infection can cause lasting damage to brain or nearby structures. Poliomyelitis may leave total paralysis or no more than a slight disability. Luckily, poliomyelitis and rabies can both be prevented by immunization.

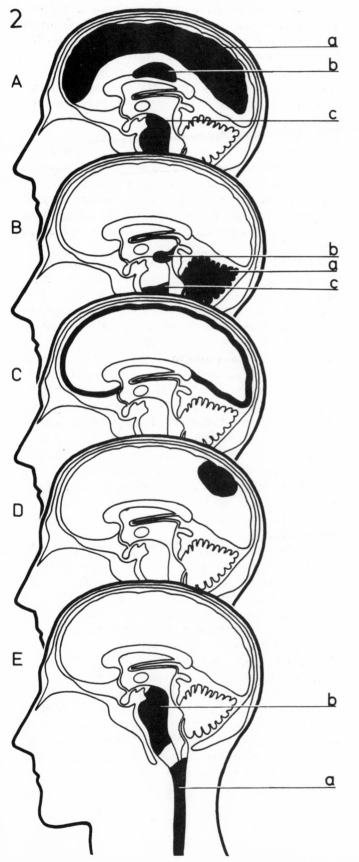

2 Brain Infections

A Encephalitis. The encephalitis virus infects and inflames large areas of the cerebral cortex (**a**), basal ganglia (**b**) and brainstem (**c**). Many neurons throughout the brain may be killed.

B Rabies. The rabies virus invades the cerebellum (**a**), hippocampus (**b**) and medulla (**c**). The resulting hydrophobia (fear of water) may be so intense that the sufferer is unable to swallow his or her own saliva, and if this stage is reached, the disease is invariably fatal.

C Meningitis. Inflammation of the pathways of the cerebrospinal fluid is usually caused by a virus or a bacterium, although occasionally a fungus or ameba is to blame. The diagram shows inflammation of the pia mater, which is the most likely of the meninges to be affected and is the one closest to the brain.

D Polioencephalitis. The polioencephalitis virus attacks the gray matter on the surface of the brain. The diagram shows a detail of the infected cerebral cortex.

E Poliomyelitis. The poliomyelitis virus grows in and ultimately kills motor neurons in the spinal cord (**a**) and brainstem (**b**), resulting in often severe paralysis. The cross-section of an infected spinal cord shows the degenerating gray matter in the area where the motor neurons leave the cord.

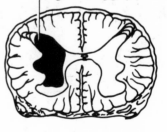

Pia mater

Infected area

Degenerating gray matter

©DIAGRAM

Injury

Head injuries are one of the commonest of all serious accidents today. Severe brain damage can kill, or turn the victim into a "vegetable." Minor injury leaves no lasting trace. Between these extremes come grades of mental and physical disability depending on the site and depth of the injury.

Many injuries produce bleeding that affects the brain. The victim may suffer headache, nausea and vomiting, and possibly lose consciousness. Speaking, and moving parts of the body, may prove difficult, and the person may feel drowsy, even falling into coma. The trouble can be due to blood collecting inside the skull and pressing on the brain. Bleeding above the dura mater – the brain's tough outer covering – produces a blood clot called an extradural hematoma. Bleeding beneath the dura causes a subdural hematoma. Left untended, either may grow large enough to leave lasting damage in the brain. Often, surgeons operate successfully. For instance, to remove a subdural clot they simply drill a hole into the skull, suck out the clot and tie off the leaking artery responsible.

Brain injuries fall into three main types: jarring, bruising and tearing – technically called concussion, contusion and laceration. Concussion is the commonest and mildest kind of brain injury. Concussed individuals may briefly go unconscious. Headaches, fatigue and insomnia are usual symptoms. Memory and some other higher functions of the brain may be temporarily affected.

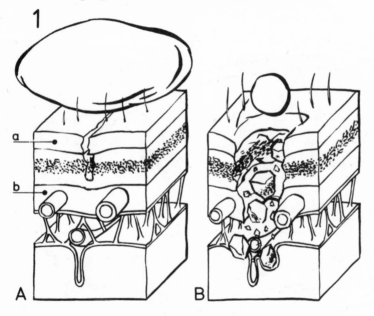

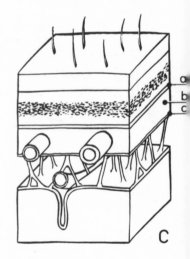

1 Skull fracture
A large stone hitting the head causes less damage than a small one.

A A large stone fractures the skull (**a**), but because a large area of bone absorbs the impact, the dura mater (**b**) is not pierced.

B A small stone causes a compound fracture and fragments of bone are driven into the brain.

C A blow on the head that causes blood to leak from an artery in the skull puts dangerous pressure on the brain. An epidural hematoma is caused by bleeding into the space (**a**) above the dura mater (**b**). A subdural hematoma is caused by blood in the space (**c**) below the dura mater.

2 Area of damage
The nerves from the right and left sides of the body cross over before they reach the motor cortex of the brain. Thus an injury to the left side of the brain causes paralysis on the right side of the body. Injuries to the top of the brain affect the feet, and injuries to areas at the base of the brain cortex affect the head and neck.

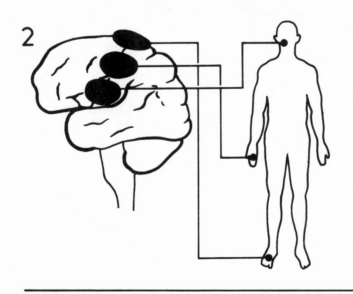

Contusion – bruising of the brain – can be more serious. The individual may lose consciousness, and this state may last for several days. If higher centers of the brain cease to function properly, subsidiary centers that they usually supervise may be affected, producing uninhibited behavior and altering the victim's personality.

Laceration is tearing of the brain – often by a piece of broken skull – and can diminish its blood supply. Germs entering the broken skull may cause serious brain infections, and scarred brain tissue may produce convulsive seizures starting months after the damage happened. Loss of memory (amnesia) may be severe – affecting not just the accident, but events before and after. The outcome of a head injury depends on several factors. The old, the deeply unconscious and those unable to remember anything since the event are least likely to recover well. Some people regain all their mental faculties yet not the full use of their limbs. Children prove the most resilient; badly brain-damaged children go on improving for up to five years after the disaster.

Luckily, head injuries leave few people with lasting physical and mental disabilities.

3 Brain Cage
The large veins that drain blood from the brain (right) form a sort of semirigid cage that limits the brain's movement. This helps protect the brain from blows and shocks, and the pressure of blood in the veins also helps keep it in the correct shape. The diagram (below) shows how a blow on the back of the head (**a**) makes the brain swish forward (**b**). Like a mushroom subjected to pressure on its cap, the greatest damage is to the midbrain areas (top of the mushroom stalk, **c**) where the spinal cord meets the brain, and to the poles at the front and back of the brain.

© DIAGRAM

Headaches

Almost everyone has had a headache at some time. Yet you might think it strange that headaches ever happen, when you remember that the brain which largely occupies the head is quite incapable of feeling pain. In fact headaches stem not from the brain itself but from vessels, nerves or muscles connected with the brain or scalp.

Headaches are often due to veins or arteries in or near the brain dilating, narrowing, or being pulled out of position. Thus raised blood pressure can cause headache by dilating branches of the external carotid artery. This dilation sets off reactions by pain-sensitive nerve-endings in the affected blood vessels. The outcome is a throbbing headache, perhaps accompanied by dizziness and vertigo. High-blood-pressure headaches have a similar

immediate origin to migraine, usually a one-sided affliction with a name that comes from *hemicrania* ("half the cranium"). Migraine tends to run in families. Sufferers endure periodic attacks, often heralded by colored lights or blurred vision produced as blood vessels that supply the brain go into spasm. Then the vessels dilate and the attack shifts into top gear with throbbing headache, nausea and photophobia (intolerance of light). Discovery that animal fats, chocolate, alcohol and other foods precipitate attacks in many individuals suggests their headaches may be due at least partly to a specific biochemical disturbance.

So-called migrainous neuralgia involves spasms of severe pain in the front of the head.

Psychogenic headaches often mimic migraine. But

1 Sinus Pain
Most headaches originate in tissues that are outside the skull (extracranial). Pain is often referred from these sources, such as the sinuses (below), to other regions of the head. Respiratory diseases, or allergies such as asthma which affect the pain-sensitive tissues of the nasal sinuses are commonly accompanied by severe headache. The pain is usually worst around the affected area, such as just over the eyes, but is often felt round the forehead and temples as well.

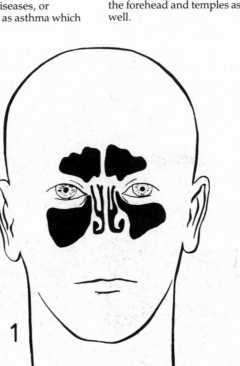

1

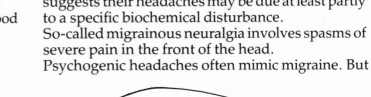

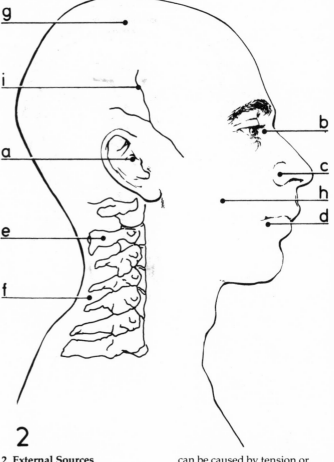

2

2 External Sources
Pain may be referred to the head from damaged or infected tissues in the ears (**a**), eyes (**b**), nose (**c**), teeth and mouth (**d**), or even, as in arthritis, areas as distant as the spinal vertebrae (**e**). Painful prolonged contraction of the muscles of the neck (**f**), scalp (**g**) and face (**h**) can be caused by tension or fatigue, or may be the result of preexisting headache affecting muscles round the head. Dilation of the arteries, particularly the temporal artery (**i**), tends to cause the throbbing nauseous pain associated with migraine.

sufferers frequently describe a "tight band" around the head due to nothing more than persistent contraction of scalp and other muscles caused by nervous stress.

Brain infections, tumors, scalp injuries and internal bleeding in the cranium can all cause headaches by affecting the pain sensors in the sheaths wrapped around the brain. Tumors probably provoke headaches less by pressing on other structures than by pulling on cerebral vessels. Infections involving ears, teeth and sinuses – hollows in the front of the skull connecting with the nostrils – any of these may unleash pain in head or face. (Incidentally, few headaches are so unendurable as the facial pain meted out by trigeminal neuralgia, a pain caused by misfunctions of the fifth cranial nerve.) Fortunately most headaches simply go away or can be treated. Painkilling drugs like aspirin relieve the "stress headaches" from which so many people suffer, and migraine often responds to ergotamine, a drug that relieves painful blood vessels.

Rarely, surgery may be required, if the headache is produced by something serious like a brain tumor, or bleeding beneath the skull.

Different types of headache have individual features that aid identification. Differences are in type of pain, time of onset, duration, frequency, and area of head affected, as well as associated symptoms such as nausea, vertigo and visual disturbance.

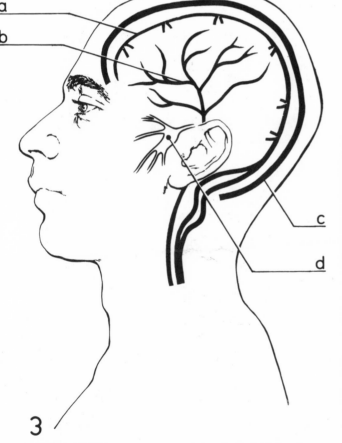

3 Internal Sources
Pain-sensitive tissues in contact with the brain include the great veins on the surface of the brain (**a**), the cerebral arteries (**b**) and parts of the dura, particularly at the base of the skull (**c**). Headache results if these are pulled or distorted as by a tumor or hemorrhage, or if the areas around them become inflamed as with infections like meningitis. Pain may also result from irritation or pressure on nerves such as the trigeminal (**d**) that have their roots in the brain.

4 Migraine
Many people experience similar sensations of bright lights at the onset of a migraine attack. The lights typically form characteristic patterns (fortification patterns) of which the c-shaped grouping of bars of light is the most common. The sensation is due to groups of neurons in the visual cortex firing together. This, in turn, is thought to be caused by the contraction of cerebral arteries which cuts off the supply of oxygen to some areas of the brain.

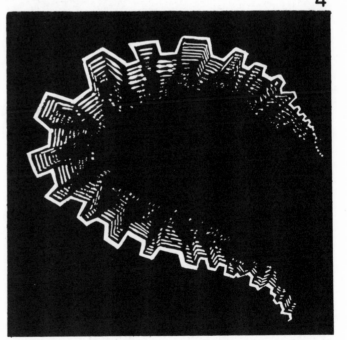

©DIAGRAM

Epilepsy

Epilepsy means "seizure." Epileptics suffer repeated fits or other seizures when electrical storms rage through the brain. No fewer than two million Americans live with this neurological handicap – more than suffer any other except stroke.

Epilepsy takes many forms, now internationally grouped in two main types: generalized attacks and those termed focal, partial or localized. Some start in one part of the brain and invade others. Generalized convulsive attacks (alias grand mal or tonic-clonic attacks) account for over half of all fits. Many start with an aura: an unpleasant sensation or a strange smell, taste, sound or vision produced by the part of the brain where the trouble begins. As trouble spreads through the brain, more parts stop working properly, so more of the body goes out of control. The victim falls down unconscious. For moments, his body lies stiff, often with outstretched limbs. Then these make short, jerky movements. The person may bite his tongue, foam at the mouth, and urinate. The attack subsides as the brain's overexcited neurons grow exhausted. Unconsciousness gives way to sleep, or confused consciousness. When normal consciousness returns, perhaps hours later, the individual cannot recall what happened.

1 Firing Neurons
Neurons in the brain are continuously firing in often recognizable patterns.
A Some neurons in the cerebral cortex produce regular, widely spaced impulses.
B Other neurons fire much more irregularly, producing a few closely spaced impulses at irregular intervals.
C Epileptic neurons typically produce groups of extremely closely spaced impulses in fairly regular bursts.

2 Brain Waves
a A normal pattern of alpha waves in a relaxed person.
b In a petit mal epileptic fit there is a regular alternation of a large rapid upward spike and a slower downward recovery one.
c In a grand mal epileptic fit, random large slow waves (delta waves) predominate as many of the neurons in the brain cortex fire simultaneously.

3 Noise-Induced Epilepsy
A particular sound may induce an epileptic fit in a susceptible person. In one person, the sound of bells started off strong rhythms in previously inactive neurons in the temporal cortex. After 22 seconds the rhythms had spread to 6 out of the 8 parts of the brain under investigation, and a fit resulted.

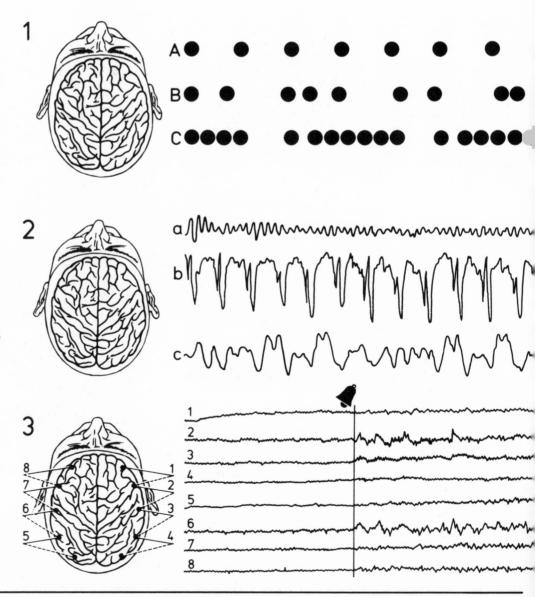

Temporal-lobe epilepsy (with attacks that arise in the brain's temporal lobes) is the next commonest form. Victims experience memory upsets and vivid hallucinations of things smelled, tasted, heard or seen. Some saints' visions may have occurred in this way. Rather than falling down, patients may briefly become automatons, perhaps even undressing in some public place.

Lesser kinds of epilepsy include petit mal ("little sickness") where the person momentarily "freezes;" and drop attacks, where the victim falls with no warning, and gets up at once.

The extent and nature·of an epileptic attack hold clues to the area or areas of brain affected. The cause may be more difficult to find. But brain scans and other diagnostic aids now help doctors to differentiate between an inherited tendency to fits and those due to brain tumors, head injuries, brain infections and other causes. Incidentally, some "fits" turn out to be no more than hysteria, fainting or breath-holding.

Treatment depends upon the type of epilepsy. Sometimes removing an affected bit of brain cures the trouble. But most patients find that taking anticonvulsant drugs prevents attacks. In fact these drugs now enable more than four-fifths of all epileptics to lead normal lives.

4 Light-Induced Epilepsy
A flashing light, even the flicker of a television picture, can produce an epileptic fit. The diagram shows how a rapidly flashing light shone into a person's eyes for a short period stimulated a massive discharge of electrical activity in the brain. Neurons from all areas of the cortex fired together at a low frequency – the typical pattern of epilepsy.

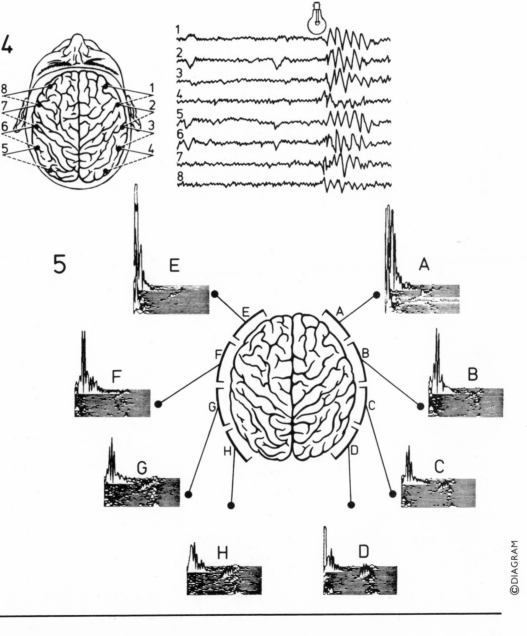

5 Compressed Spectral Array
This is an advanced computerized method for pictorially representing the electrical activity occurring simultaneously in different parts of the brain. Each of the 8 diagrams represents an area of the cerebral cortex of an epileptic person stimulated by a flashing light. The peaks show the firing of neurons in each of these areas. The large spikes to the left of each diagram are abnormal discharges that can be correlated with the actual behavior of neurons during an epileptic fit. A close study of the diagrams shows that the epileptic discharges are triggered slightly earlier in the front parts of the brain (**A** and **E**) than in the sides and rear.

©DIAGRAM

137

Tumors

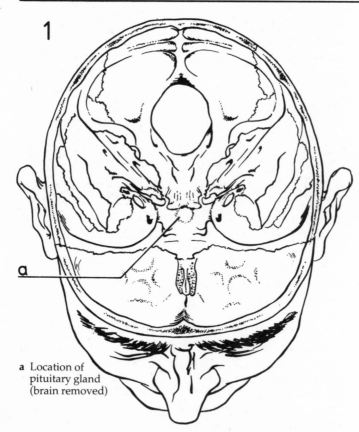

1

a Location of pituitary gland (brain removed)

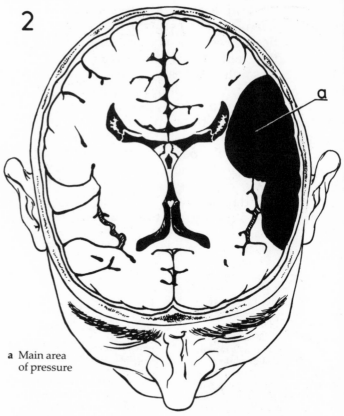

2

a Main area of pressure

1 Pituitary Tumor
A pituitary tumor may be small and slow growing, but the effects can be drastic. The tumor interferes with the normal production of hormones, so hormone levels either fall or increase enormously. Massive overproduction of pituitary hormones can result in a form of giantism (acromegaly) in which the hands, face and feet become grossly increased in size. Too low a level of some pituitary hormones can cause dwarfism or diabetes insipidus. Only a small change in hormone levels is needed to upset completely essential body functions such as metabolism.

2 Meningioma
A tumor of the meninges (a meningioma) is typically slow growing but may prove fatal because of the pressure it exerts on the brain. As with any brain damage, the effects of pressure vary according to the area of the brain that becomes distorted. A meningioma that presses on the left temporal lobe (as in the diagram) would, if unchecked, result in impairment of speech and understanding. As the tumor grows, more areas become distorted and greater pressure is set up. Commonly, a meningioma will cause distortion of the cavities containing cerebrospinal fluid. This results in blockage of the flow and a build-up of fluid, which itself causes even greater pressure.

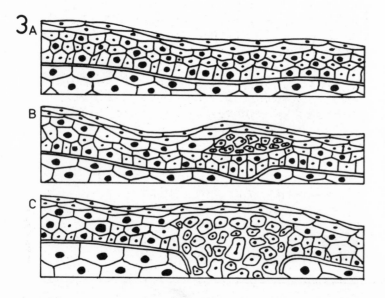

3A

B

C

3 Malignant Growth
Unlike a benign tumor which grows slowly, the cells of a malignant tumor (a cancer) spread rapidly and uncontrollably.
A In normal tissue, cells are arranged in an orderly manner and divide to form new cells with the same characteristics and functions as the surrounding tissue.

B A mutant cell or a cancer cell from another part of the body starts dividing more rapidly than the surrounding cells, and begins to form a growth that markedly differs from the original tissue.
C As the cells continue to divide haphazardly, the tumor spreads until it dominates and finally replaces the original tissue. Unchecked, the tumor will grow to fill all available space.

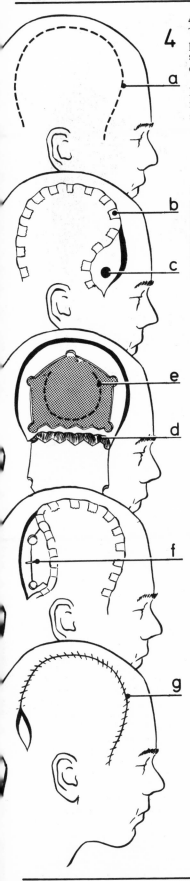

4 Pressure Relief
The only way to relieve the pressure caused by a tumor is by surgical removal of all or some of the tumor.

First, a semicircular incision (**a**) is made through the flesh of the scalp.

Clamps (**b**) are applied to the cut edge of the skin, which is pulled back to expose the skull bone. Holes (**c**) are drilled through this at intervals of 4cm along the length of the incision, and the bone between them is sawn through.

Now the whole flap of bone and scalp can be pulled outward, using the jaw muscles (**d**) at its base as a hinge. The dura mater (**e**) is cut through with scissors to reveal the surface of the brain.

After removing the tumor, the bone flap is replaced and held tightly against the rest of the skull by wire sutures (**f**).

The clamps are removed and the surface of the scalp is sutured together with fine silk thread (**g**).

Tumors – abnormal growths – can occur inside the brain itself or in its coverings beneath the skull. Because the skull cannot readily expand to make room for a growing tumor, this presses on the brain and causes damage that may lead to death if left untreated.

Various types of cell multiplying uncontrolled can create tumors inside the cranium. Some sprout from cancer cells that have migrated from another region of the body. Some tumors that originate inside the cranium are not produced by brain cells. These can arise from the blood vessels that supply the brain, from the meningeal sheaths that cover it, or from the pituitary gland inside it. However, most tumors are gliomas – so-called because they start in the glial ("glue") cells that support the neurons. Brain tumors rarely develop in the neurons themselves – the cells that all brain activity directly depends upon.

Certain tumors grow faster than others. Some benign tumors expand so slowly they may take years becoming a noticeable nuisance. On the other hand a malignant tumor may grow fast enough to change the brain fatally in months. Signs and symptoms often stem from pressure set up in the skull, especially when a tumor blocks cerebrospinal fluid flow so that liquid swells the cavities in the brain. Headaches, blurred vision, nausea and vomiting may all be brought on by a tumor of the brain (as well, of course, as by far less serious conditions). Eventually a growing tumor also interferes with the normal working of the region of the brain affected. Smell, speech, touch perception, movement of one side of the body, mental powers – any one of these faculties or others may become impaired. Also, many patients suffer convulsions similar to epileptic fits.

Modern brain-scanning devices or other diagnostic aids often make it easy to detect and localize a tumor. The next step, if possible, is operating to remove it. Sometimes the surgeon may have to cut a semicircle in the skull and raise this bony flap to reach the brain beneath. Using a blunt cutting instrument, he removes diseased tissue, taking care not to tamper with the motor cortex, for that might leave the patient speechless and paralyzed or weak down one side. Often surgery can totally remove noninvasive – nonmalignant – tumors such as meningiomas, and partial removal of malignant tumors can relieve pressure on the brain. Deep tumors can be attacked with X-rays, probes, or cauterizing needles to destroy as much of the diseased tissue as possible.

© DIAGRAM

Strokes

The word "stroke" suggests a sudden blow. Often, but not always, that is how strokes strike down their victims. The cause is brain damage due to blood blockage or leakage. More men than women suffer strokes, and over 60 is the most vulnerable age. All told, 2.5 million Americans (1.1 per cent of the population) have had their lives impaired by these so-called cerebrovascular accidents.

Strokes come in three main kinds. In cerebral hemorrhage, a blood vessel bursts in the brain, and the heart's pumping action squirts blood into brain tissue, producing a clot that kills cells and maybe presses on the brainstem. Brain hemorrhage may happen if one of the brain's blood vessels (among the body's weakest) gets brittle, and bursts under abnormally high blood pressure, or when a weak spot in the wall of a vessel balloons out and bursts like a defective tire wall.

Strokes are also caused by cerebral thrombosis and cerebral embolus. In cerebral thrombosis, local clogging up of a blood vessel produces a thrombus (clot) blocking the vessel. The brain is denied glucose and oxygen usually supplied by that vessel; brain cells deprived in this way quickly die and cannot be replaced. The same thing happens with cerebral embolus ("plug"). A plug of material that had been circulating through the bloodstream gets stuck in a narrowed blood vessel. In fact most strokes happen when a clot blocks a cerebral artery.

Symptoms of a stroke range from brief confusion, dizziness or slurred speech (a transient ischemic attack, where a blood vessel is only temporarily blocked) to throbbing headache, vomiting,

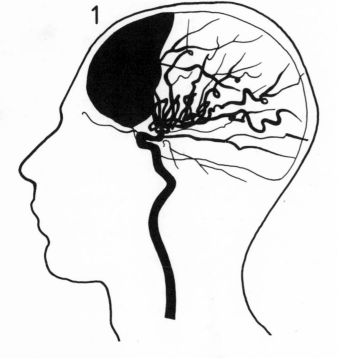

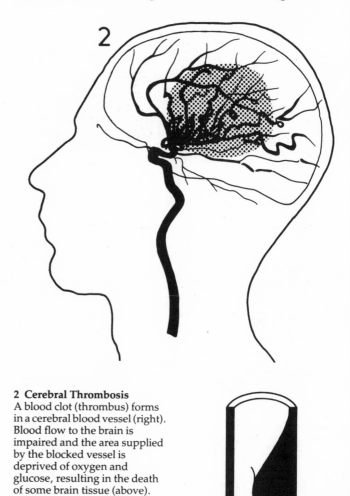

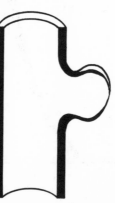

1 Cerebral Hemorrhage
A weak or diseased spot in the wall of a blood vessel swells out and ruptures (right). Blood from the damaged area floods into the surrounding brain tissue and clots. The clot enlarges, as shown above, as blood continues to pour in, and eventually presses on the brain.

2 Cerebral Thrombosis
A blood clot (thrombus) forms in a cerebral blood vessel (right). Blood flow to the brain is impaired and the area supplied by the blocked vessel is deprived of oxygen and glucose, resulting in the death of some brain tissue (above).

numbness of limbs, partial paralysis, or coma. Damage done depends on the part and amount of brain affected. A huge fast-growing clot pressing on the brain, or swelling due to the death of many brain cells, affects the brainstem, causing coma and death if not quickly treated. Blockage of the right middle cerebral artery may produce a massive so-called "President's stroke" paralyzing the left side of the body. Yet if brain damage affects only part of the right parietal lobe, the patient may seem normal except for visuospatial problems, for instance thrusting an arm in a pants leg when dressing. But strokes often affect gait, hearing, speech or vision.

Luckily, treatment for stroke victims has vastly improved. CAT scans, X-ray angiograms that make blood vessels "glow" and other tests help surgeons to identify and localize damage. Aided by microscopes, microneedles and microsutures they can often clear clots or use a synthetic blood vessel to bypass a blocked internal carotid artery. Drugs also have parts to play: controlling blood clotting; lowering high blood pressure; or, with vasodilators, expanding blood vessels to prevent major strokes in patients who have had transient ischemic episodes.

After someone has survived a serious stroke, physiotherapy can often do much to prevent deformities such as foot drop. Also, signals blocked by a damaged neuron circuit may be rerouted eventually through others, so that the patient slowly recovers lost faculties. The extent of recovery varies with age, health and the type of damage the brain has sustained.

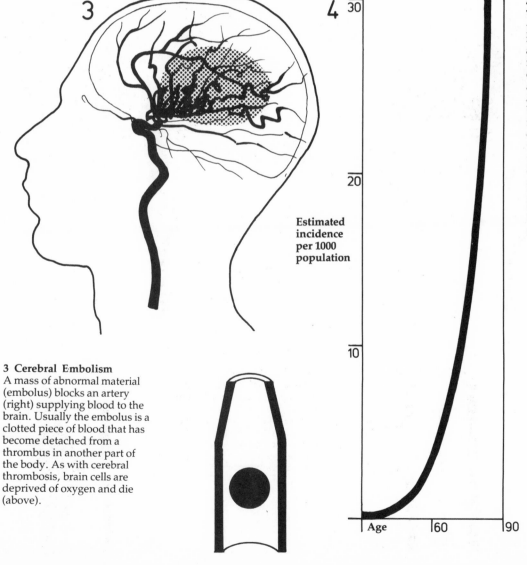

Estimated incidence per 1000 population

3 Cerebral Embolism
A mass of abnormal material (embolus) blocks an artery (right) supplying blood to the brain. Usually the embolus is a clotted piece of blood that has become detached from a thrombus in another part of the body. As with cerebral thrombosis, brain cells are deprived of oxygen and die (above).

4 Incidence of Strokes
The graph shows that the probability of having a stroke increases with age. This is partly a result of the rapidly increasing incidence of arterial disease, especially hardening of the arteries (arteriosclerosis), with age. Arteriosclerosis leads to the build up of clotted blood on the inner walls of the arteries and eventually the formation of a thrombus. High blood pressure, a condition also common amongst older people, adds to the danger of a stroke both by making the rupture of a brain artery more likely and because of its association with arterial disease.

©DIAGRAM

Degenerative Diseases

Degenerative diseases affecting the brain range from the swiftly fatal to some that may produce only slight disability after many years. New understanding of brain chemistry now relieves symptoms in thousands of patients.

Multiple sclerosis (literally, "multiple scars") alias disseminated sclerosis, is a disease that destroys in seemingly random fashion the myelin sheaths that help axons conduct signals from one neuron to another. The brain's white matter, optic nerves and spinal cord can all be affected. Victims may first notice loss of vision in one eye, or partial paralysis. The symptoms may go, but others appear later, perhaps with eventual incapacity and other interference with brain function. Young adults are those most often hit. However, many patients remain active for years – some for decades. ACTH or steroids relieve acute inflammatory attacks, but life expectancy is shortened in most cases.

Between the ages 30 and 45 some 6 people per 100,000 develop Huntington's chorea ("dance"). Degeneration of cerebrum and basal ganglia cause involuntary movements of face, body, hands and feet, and victims of this rare, hereditary affliction usually die in mental hospitals.

Over 50's are likeliest to contract motor-neuron disease, an especially unpleasant condition that attacks neurons which operate muscles. Speech or swallowing may become difficult, and there may be wasting and weakness in muscles of the tongue, hands, and later other parts of the body. Twice as many men as women contract motor-neuron disease, for which there is as yet no satisfactory treatment.

First described in 1817 by James Parkinson,

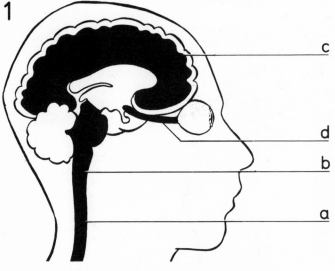

1

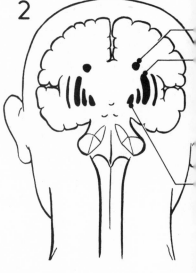

2

2 Huntington's Chorea
This rare, invariably fatal, hereditary disease resembles accelerated aging. It is associated with degeneration of nerve tissue in the basal ganglia – particularly the caudate nucleus (**a**) and putamen (**b**), and occasionally the globus pallidus (**c**).
Sufferers develop spasmodic movements, speech difficulties, and psychological disorders leading eventually to dementia. Huntington's chorea is transmitted by an abnormal dominant gene. The diagram (below) shows how only one parent need possess this gene for 1 in 2 children to be at risk. By the time the disease develops – sometimes only in a person's 50s or 60s – an affected person may have grandchildren with a 50:50 chance of developing the disease.

1 Multiple Sclerosis
This is a disease caused by an unknown agent, possibly a virus, that attacks myelinated nerves. Nerves of the spinal cord (**a**), brainstem (**b**), cerebral hemispheres (**c**) and the optic nerve (**d**) may all be affected. In a diseased nerve (right), the myelin sheath (**A**) surrounding the axon (**B**) begins to erode. Hard (sclerotic) patches form, resulting in the interruption of nerve impulses, particularly in pathways concerned with vision, sensation and the use of limbs. Early symptoms may include temporary loss of vision or double vision, unsteadiness in walking, and dizziness. Eventually the disease results in permanent paralysis.

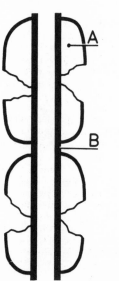

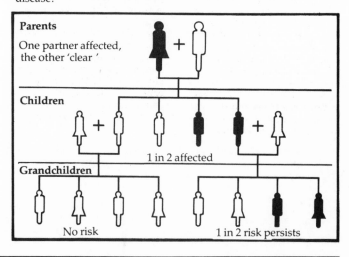

Parents
One partner affected, the other 'clear'

Children

1 in 2 affected

Grandchildren

No risk   1 in 2 risk persists

Parkinson's disease attacks mainly people aged 50 to 75, causing shaking limbs, shuffling steps, and poor balance. The face becomes blank; with staring eyes. Handwriting gets small and cramped, and fastening buttons may become difficult. The disease is progressive but affects some patients only slightly for many years.

The immediate cause is degeneration of dark cells in the substantia nigra ("black substance") in the brainstem. These are major producers of the neurotransmitter dopamine, whose absence produces rigidity and tremor. Luckily, symptoms can now be relieved and life prolonged by giving anticholinergics and L-dopa, a substance that is taken up by the brain and there converted to dopamine.

The quest for a true cure at last offers a glimmering of hope. Researchers grafting brain tissue from normal rat fetuses into the brains of rats with Parkinson-like symptoms found that some grafts successfully took and improved the patients' conditions. This suggests that one day there may be a role for human brain grafts too. In 1981 other workers suggested stimulating the body to make dopamine by giving doses of synthetically made pterins – natural chemical agents that help to persuade amino acids to form neurotransmitters. In old age (sometimes earlier) brain atrophy due to impaired blood supply may impair mental faculties, producing Alzheimer's dementia, in which patients become unable to think or remember, and selfish emotions override judgment. As senile dementia progresses, the brain's highest, most recently evolved, centers stop working first. Last to go is the brainstem – the most primitive part of the brain.

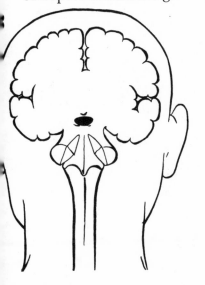
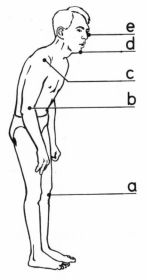
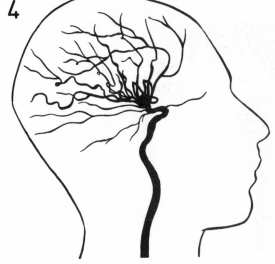

3 Parkinson's Disease

Parkinsonism (paralysis agitans) is another disease of the basal ganglia, especially the substantia nigra (shown above). The disease, which affects voluntary motor nerves, results in slowness and loss of movement (akinesia), muscular rigidity, and tremor which may at first be localized but spreads to many muscles as the disease progresses. Speech difficulties (dysarthria) and inability to perform everyday activities like washing and dressing may be experienced. The sufferer develops a characteristic stance (above) with the knees (**a**) and elbows (**b**) slightly bent, the shoulders stooping (**c**) and the chin sunk onto the chest (**d**). Rigidity of the facial muscles causes the face to take on a fixed, masklike expression (**e**).

4 Senile Dementia

Nerve cells do not divide, unlike most other cells in the body, so brain cells that die are never replaced. In old age a poor blood supply often leads to cells dying off very rapidly. This results in a general lowering of intelligence and the cessation of higher functions like memory and the ability to reason. However, only a minority of old people develop Alzheimer's dementia. Poor sight and hearing are more often due to deterioration of the ears and eyes than death of brain cells. Old age is not necessarily a time of decreasing intelligence and mental activity: vocabulary and the ability to use words often carry on improving, even into extreme old age.

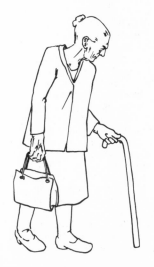

©DIAGRAM

Chapter 9

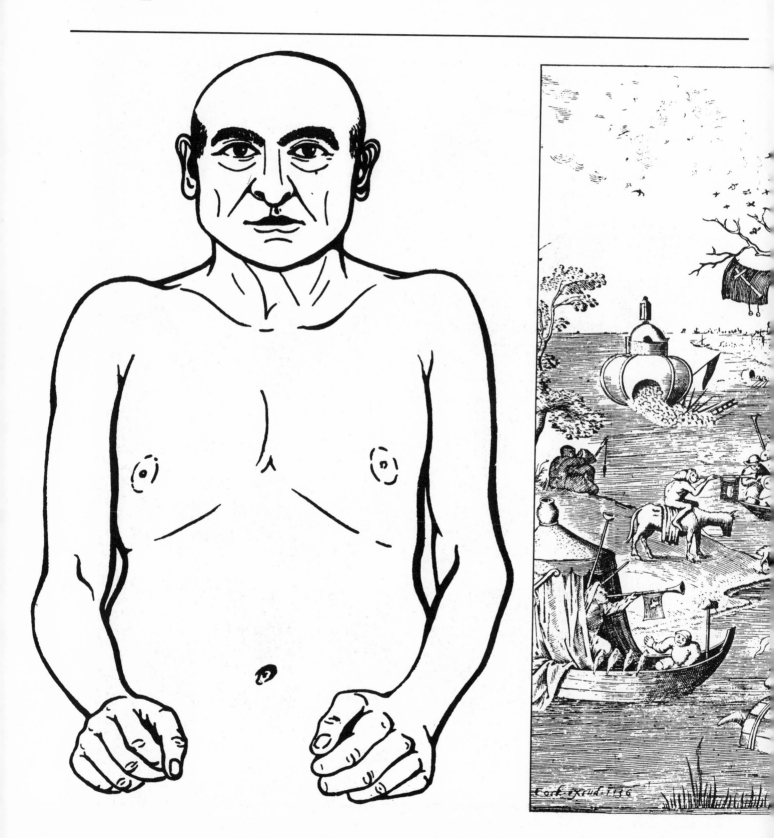

THE TROUBLED MIND

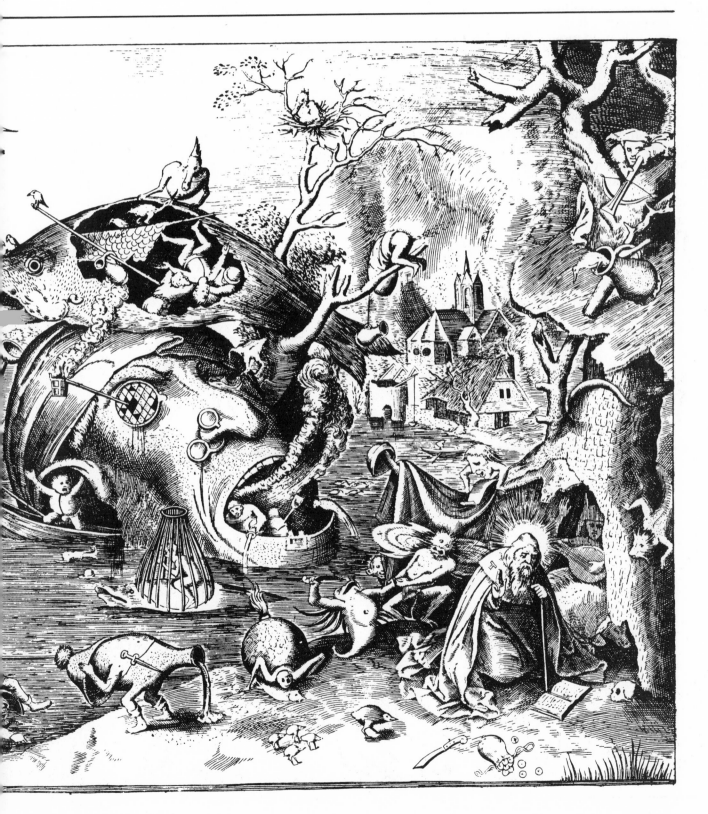

Neuroses

Some malfunctions of the mind are easily attributed to specific damage in the brain. Others are less easily pinned down. These can range from minor personality maladjustments to dangerous or incapacitating mental illness.

Neuroses come into the first, or lesser, category. These fairly mild mental disturbances sometimes feature an emotional conflict, involving a blocked impulse that finds an outlet in signs or symptoms disguising their true origin.

Many doctors recognize four main types of neurosis which may be described as anxiety, hysterical, obsessive-compulsive and depressive. Anxiety neurosis is the commonest, and often shows up as emotional overreaction to ordinary situations like shopping or travel. Anxiety neurosis also affects people who are generally well-adjusted but under severe pressure, or who are nervous before a public occasion. Symptoms may include breathlessness, rapid pulse, muscular tension, dilated pupils and sweating.

Hysterical neurosis takes two forms called conversion and dissociative hysteria. In the first kind, physical symptoms involving sensory or motor nerves help to damp down felt anxiety. People with conversion hysteria may be unable either to see, hear, speak or move a limb, though suffering no actual damage to the nerves involved. Dissociative hysterics escape overwhelming anxiety by stupor, loss of memory, entering a state of unreality, or aimless activity. Sleepwalking is a fairly common mild reaction. Rarely, one individual can assume several personalities. Obsessive-compulsive neurotics suffer from

1

1 Effects of Anxiety
The physical effects of anxiety neuroses can be alarming in the extreme, and often aggravate the effects of the neurosis itself. An anxiety reaction may include any or all the following physical symptoms:
a Tension migraine.
b Sweating.
c Dilated pupils.
d Pallor.
e Dry mouth.
f Vomiting.
g Breathlessness.
h Irregular or rapid heartbeat.
i Tremor.
j Heightened muscle tone.

obsessive thoughts or actions, for instance an obsessive fear of germs may make them wash their hands repeatedly.

Depressive neurotics may suffer unnaturally prolonged depression or feelings of inadequacy, guilt and hopelessness following stress involving loss. Divorce, redundancy, a failed examination, or death of a close friend or relative may start this condition. Occasionally it may disappear in time, without any special treatment.

Many neurotic people find relief in just talking over their problem with their doctor or life partner, or with a marriage guidance counselor. Some benefit best from tranquilizers, others from practical help, for instance with money problems. Behavior therapy may assist sufferers from agoraphobia (fear of open spaces) and other phobias to cope with daily fear-provoking situations. In the United States, psychotherapy is widely used against neurosis. (See page 152.)

2 Types of Neurosis

Neuroses are often classified into four main types.

a Anxiety neuroses consist of overreaction to an everyday event, such as seeing a particular animal or standing in a confined space.

b Hysterical neuroses involve the shutting down of some part of the body's system, such as one of the senses or motor control, so that the person does not have to confront the object of his fear.

c Obsessive neuroses involve inappropriate repetitions of certain thoughts or actions.

d Depressive neuroses involve inappropriately severe feelings of inadequacy in response to emotional stress or minor failures.

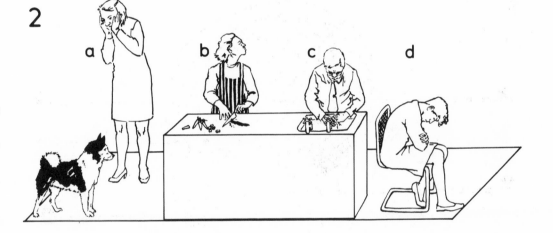

3 Phobias

Phobias can be classified into four main types: animal phobias; other specific phobias such as fear of water or of heights; social phobias such as fear of crowds or of specific types of people; and agoraphobia, fear of the outdoor world.

Psychotherapists have noted that animal phobias (**A**) tend to begin at around age 4, while the other types of phobia generally have much later onsets. Social phobias (**B**) begin at an average age of 19, other specific phobias (**C**) around age 23, and agoraphobia (**D**) at about age 24.

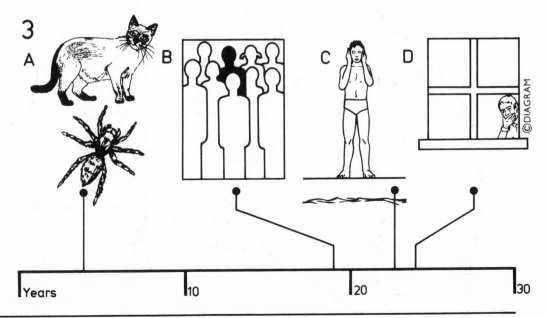

Psychoses

Psychoses are serious mental illnesses affecting the entire personality, with far more disabling effects than neurotic people suffer. The three main groups of psychoses are schizophrenia, manic depression and severe depressive illness.

Despite its name, schizophrenia ("split mind") does not involve the multiple personalities found in one form of hysteria. Rather, the personality disintegrates, and there is loss of contact with reality. Schizophrenics often show a lack of appropriate emotional response, suspect people of hostility, and hide their real feelings. They may express a string of unconnected thoughts, and experience opposite feelings simultaneously toward some other person. They may even behave autistically, thinking in a self-centered way, daydreaming, fantasizing, and attributing unusual meanings to certain words.

Schizophrenics make up one quarter of all state mental hospital admissions and take up half the beds available because many respond less readily to treatment than some other mental patients. Manic depressives suffer attacks involving violent mood swings. The manic phase is one of active optimism, when the individual forms exciting plans that grow more grandiose and less well reasoned as the phase advances. A manic person may go on spending sprees, phone slight acquaintances at night, and seek legal action against people in authority who try to balk him. The depressive phase is marked by sadness, guilt, perhaps delusions, slowed movements and delayed reactions in conversation. The patient is now aware of his condition and may try suicide.

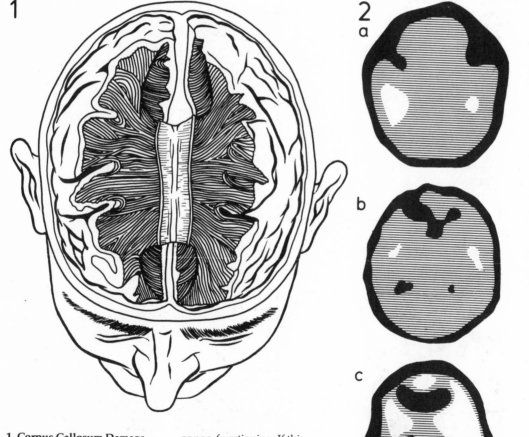

1

2

a

b

c

2 Brain Scans
PETT scans (see pp. 122–123) used in tests on schizophrenics and manic-depressives in New York have revealed abnormalities in the brain's glucose consumption. The scans of schizophrenic patients showed decreased glucose consumption in some areas, while scans of manic-depressives showed increased consumption during the manic phases of their symptoms. Similar scans may enable neurologists to diagnose these confusing mental illnesses with greater accuracy in the future.
a Scan showing normal glucose consumption.
b Scan of schizophrenic.
c Scan of manic-depressive.

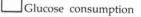 Glucose consumption

1 Corpus Callosum Damage
Recent research into schizophrenia has suggested that some sufferers may have abnormalities of the corpus callosum, the bridge between the two halves of the brain. Scans and other tests on a small number of schizophrenics have revealed that each corpus callosum is thickened, damaged or non-functioning. If this proved to be the case with most schizophrenics it would perhaps be possible in the future to provide screening before schizophrenic symptoms occur, so that preventative treatment could be given.

Some people suffer from severe depression, often after a stressful event such as giving birth, the menopause, retirement, redundancy, death of a parent, or departure from home of a grown-up child. At first the patient may sleep badly, grow irritable, and worry. As depression deepens, there may be a sense of guilt, delusions, agitation – many patients often wring their hands – and even plans of suicide.

Until recently, there seemed no logical explanation for conditions like those that we have just described. Increasingly, however, doctors are blaming them on brain-chemistry malfunction. It is suggested that drugs reducing the active amount of the neurotransmitter norepinephrine induce depression, while drugs increasing the amount help to raise a patient's spirits. Doctors think that

schizophrenia coincides with too much of the neurotransmitter dopamine in the brain's limbic system, and counter this with drug antagonists of dopamine, often so successfully that many a schizophrenic can take a rehabilitation course, return from hospital, and even work again.

It is also thought that long-term use of lithium carbonate helps to prevent the extreme mood swings found in manic depression. The last pages in this chapter examine in more detail the use of drugs and other aids in treating mental illness.

3 Severe Depression

As its name suggests, this illness is a more severe and debilitating version of the common phases of depression through which most people pass unscathed. In susceptible people, however, the depression deepens until it can be recognized as a true illness rather than a passing phase, and requires treatment as soon as possible. Situations involving emotional stress often act as catalysts in the development of severe depression.

a Postnatal depression may be mild or severe.

b The death of a spouse or close relative is extremely stressful.

c The emotional and social upheaval of divorce may lead to severe depression.

d Retirement can be a severe shock to the system of career-minded people.

4 Care of the Mentally Ill

The bar (right) shows in diagrammatic form the breakdown of expenditure in the United States on direct care of the mentally ill. Types of care offered include ordinary treatment from general practitioners, drug therapy, and admissions and outpatient treatment in psychiatric hospitals.

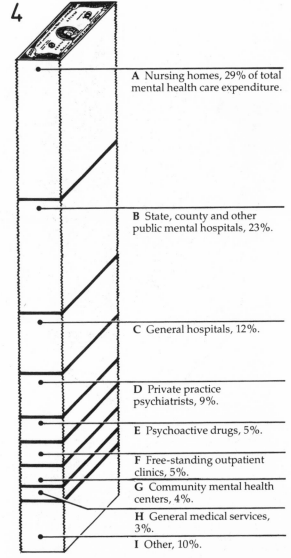

A Nursing homes, 29% of total mental health care expenditure.

B State, county and other public mental hospitals, 23%.

C General hospitals, 12%.

D Private practice psychiatrists, 9%.

E Psychoactive drugs, 5%.

F Free-standing outpatient clinics, 5%.

G Community mental health centers, 4%.

H General medical services, 3%.

I Other, 10%.

© DIAGRAM

Mind-Made Ailments

The mind is capable of engineering real or imagined ailments affecting regions of the body far beyond the brain.

Hypochondriacs – people morbidly preoccupied with their health – may misinterpret normal signals to the brain from the sensory receptors deep inside the body. Such people may complain of weakness, tiredness, imagined headaches, backache, and unexplained pains in face and abdomen. Sometimes, though, over- or understimulation of sense organs provokes changes in hormone output affecting various body systems. In turn, these changes may cause inner sensory receptors to send faulty signals to the brain, causing it to dispatch misguided instructions. The consequence may be a rapid heartbeat, palpitations, fainting, overbreathing, increased or decreased

contractions of muscles in the stomach and intestines, or muscle pains. All this can happen without giving rise to actual bodily disease. Real physical disorders brought on or worsened by emotional stress are called psychosomatic illnesses. Sometimes stress affects digestive, respiratory or other organs in ways that help to trigger asthma, high blood pressure, peptic ulcers, ulcerative colitis, or a skin disease. Doctors studying mentally induced illness think that mental stress depresses metabolism and impairs the body's immune system, making people liable to a whole host of troubles ranging from colds and influenza to heart disease and cancer. Research suggests that the risk of psychosomatic illness is greatest among those suffering from a build-up of adverse "life-events" such as job loss,

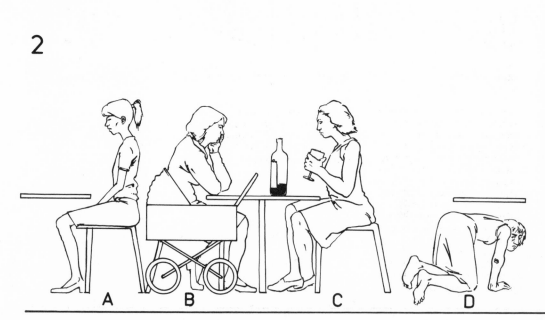

1 Effects of Stress
Stress has been shown to contribute to, or aggravate, physical disorders such as:
a Headache.
b Exhaustion.
c Excessive sweating.
d Facial flushing.
e Nasal catarrh.
f Asthma attacks.
g High blood pressure.
h Heart disease.
i Skin disease.
j Stomach problems.
k Vague aches and pains.
l Diabetes.
m Diarrhea.
n Rheumatism and arthritis.

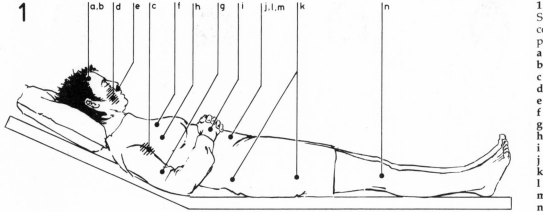

2 Psychological Effects of Stress
Prolonged periods of stress may cause, or precipitate, mental illness which may manifest itself in a variety of ways.
A Attempts to escape from a stressful lifestyle may result in neuroses or phobias, while a stressed family background may be associated with schizophrenia.
B Postnatal depression affects mothers at a time when everyone around expects them to be overjoyed. The exact causes are not yet understood.
C Individuals suffering stress may resort to excessive drinking, or to use of drugs, as a means of escape.
D Prolonged stress may result in complete withdrawal, or in irrational behavior such as outbursts of violence.

change of occupation, retirement, divorce, and death or major illness in the family. One survey showed that risk of illness increases sharply in individuals suffering more than a certain number of life events in just one year. Seemingly their cumulative effects overtax the brain's ability to adapt to hostile change.

Job loss – an all-too-common life event these days – illustrates what sometimes happens. In work, the individual could channel creative drives, feel pride in achievement, enjoy self esteem. Redundancy triggers three phases of psychological response: (1) shock and denial briefly followed by optimism; (2) mounting distress, depression and family quarrels, if job-seeking fails; (3) resignation, hopelessness and sense of failure. One study of long-term unemployment showed a rise in blood pressure and other adverse circulation changes that coincided with depression setting in with expected redundancy, and remained until the people found new jobs.

Anorexia nervosa ("nervous loss of appetite") is an unusual psychosomatic condition occurring in some teenage girls, maybe stressed by anxiety about their work and physical development. Sufferers diet so severely that they grow emaciated and cease menstruating, yet remain restlessly active and maintain they are too fat.

Many psychosomatic conditions benefit from treatments that control neuroses, and some doctors favor so-called autogenic training.

3

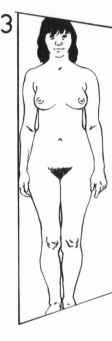 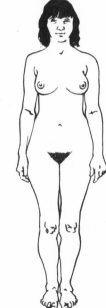 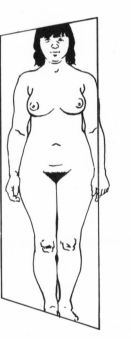 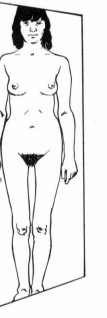 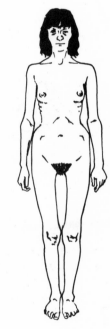

| Normal reflection | Average-sized girl | Anorectic reflection | Anorectic reflection | Chronic anorectic |

3 Anorexia Nervosa

This condition is one of the most severe psychosomatic disorders, as it can be fatal if untreated. Adolescent girls, often worried about the changes rapidly occurring in their bodies (and often simultaneously under severe academic pressure at school), embark on rigorous reducing diets or simply stop eating altogether. The condition is characterized by assertions from the sufferer that she is fat, even when she is quite obviously emaciated and starving. Anorectics appear to have a distorted view of their own body shape, overestimating their body measurements and depicting themselves graphically as being much fatter than they truly are. The severe physical effects of prolonged self-starvation include the following: sleep disturbance; excessive fatigue; hypothermia; hormone imbalance; chronic constipation; amenorrhea (cessation of menstruation); growth of excess body hair; reductions in pulse rate, respiration rate and blood pressure; and dangerous alterations in the body's electrolyte balance.

©DIAGRAM

Psychotherapy

Psychotherapy – the care and cure of the mind – uses psychological rather than surgical or ordinary medical means to treat people suffering from emotional or mental problems. There are more than 250 kinds of psychotherapeutic treatment. Best known is psychoanalysis, based on discoveries by the nineteeth-century Austrian doctor Sigmund Freud. The patient relaxes on a couch and the therapist (usually a psychiatrist) sits behind him, out of sight. The patient tells the therapist all random memories and thoughts entering his mind – a process known as free association. By gradually bringing to the surface unconscious thoughts and wishes, this technique helps the therapist discover and resolve mental conflicts caused by repressing childhood desires. At first, patients usually resist telling all, and a course of treatment to reconstruct a badly damaged personality may involve three or four sessions a week for several years.

Freudian theory influenced the now popular transactional analysis and rebirthing therapies. In the first, patients see their feelings, thoughts and behavior originating in child, adult, parent – three rival personalities in one mind. "Rebirthers" blame neuroses on birth trauma, and seek to banish their harmful effects by encouraging patients to reenact their birth. Equally dramatic is primal therapy where the therapist disturbs a patient until he gives vent to a "primal scream" releasing tension pent up by a lifelong backlog of pain. Less drastic than courses aimed at totally reconstructing personality, reeducative psychotherapies try to help patients to learn how past events influenced their present undesirable behavior patterns and how these might be modified. Therapists guide rather than direct, so that patients become self reliant. Courses involve once-weekly treatment for 9 to 18 months. Humanistic psychology, pioneered by Chicago's Carl C. Rogers, tries restoring a patient's good feelings about himself as a means to redirecting his

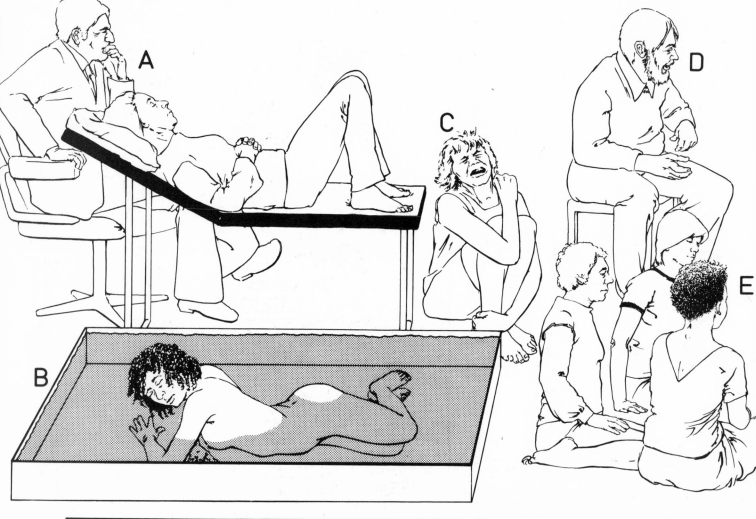

life toward fresh goals and self-fulfillment. General practitioners as well as specialists can often help with counseling to tide patients over relatively short-lived crises. Talking over current difficulties may help such patients to tackle future problems. This kind of supportive treatment usually lasts four months or less.

Because an individual's emotional problems are often closely bound up with his family, therapists often like to see life partners together. Also, patients without major personality problems may benefit as members of an encounter group. Frank verbal interchange – sometimes even stroking or hitting other members of the group – helps some people to express their feelings and gain new insight into their personalities.

Rejecting conventional psychotherapy, behaviorists try changing patients' behavior by a process of conditioning based on rewards or punishments. Yet other treatments involve hypnosis and techniques of self suggestion.

Freeing the Mind
The illustration (below) portrays some of the most widely used of the current psychotherapeutic techniques. In **A** a patient lets his thoughts roam freely while the therapist listens for clues to causes of conflict. The rebirth technique (**B**) and primal therapy (**C**) are developments of Freud's pioneering techniques. Reeducative therapy (**D**), group therapy (**E**), and family therapy (**F**) all work on the basis of a free discussion of problems in which the therapist takes a counseling role – helping the patients to understand their own emotions and problems and so come to terms with them. Self-suggestion and self-hypnosis methods (**G**) are rather more experimental but have their adherents, particularly in the United States of America.

©DIAGRAM

Calming the Troubled Mind

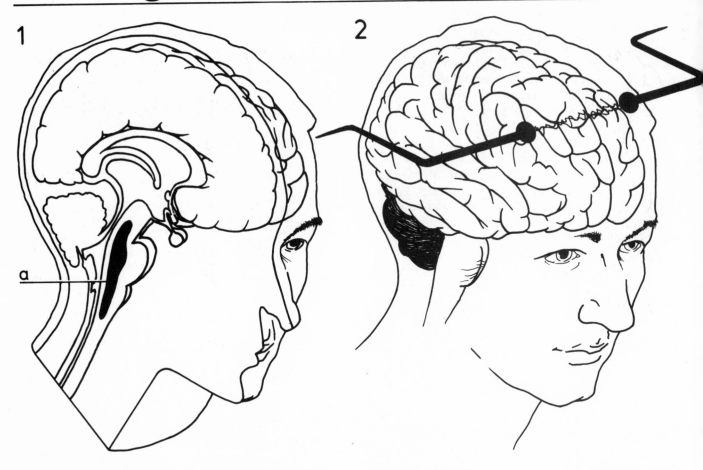

1

2

1 Psychotherapeutic Drugs
Drugs are used to treat a wide range of mental conditions as they are usually effective in alleviating symptoms. They do not always, however, help to cure the underlying illness. Most drugs work by affecting the transfer of messages between neurons – sedatives slow down the brain and so may calm patients with schizophrenia or anxiety neurosis. Some drugs affect the reticular formation (**a**), which helps to regulate consciousness and the level of activity in the rest of the brain.

2 Electroconvulsive Therapy (ECT)
Some doctors consider ECT to be helpful in the treatment of severe depression. The patient is given a drug to relax the muscles, and a general anesthetic. An electric current is then applied to the brain through electrodes taped to the scalp. This results in furious electrical activity in the brain and is similar to an epileptic fit or seizure. The patient wakens soon after and may suffer from a temporary loss of memory. The treatment is repeated over a few weeks.

Besides psychotherapy, three main weapons may be mobilized to tackle mental illness.
Most used is a battery of psychotherapeutic drugs. Major tranquilizers like chlorpromazine stop nerve-cell receptors in the brain accepting too much of the neurotransmitter dopamine. The effect is to calm schizophrenics, abolishing their hallucinations and reordering disordered thoughts. Mild tranquilizers like chlordiazepoxide (Librium) and meprobamate relieve anxiety in neurotic patients. Antidepressants such as the so-called tricyclic drug imipramine relieve depression by increasing active amounts of the neurotransmitters norepinephrine and serotonin in the brain. MAO (monamine oxidase) inhibitors achieve the same end in another way, but unwanted side-effects have reduced their popularity.
Paradoxically, stimulants like methylphenidate quieten some unmanageably hyperactive children, making them amenable to schooling. One writer claims that one million American children were being drugged like this by the middle 1970s. Many showed no benefits, and some suffered side-effects like insomnia and loss of appetite. Despite such snags – and the fact that drugs merely control mental symptoms – doctors now tend to use drugs as their first line of defense when it comes to treating many forms of mental illness.

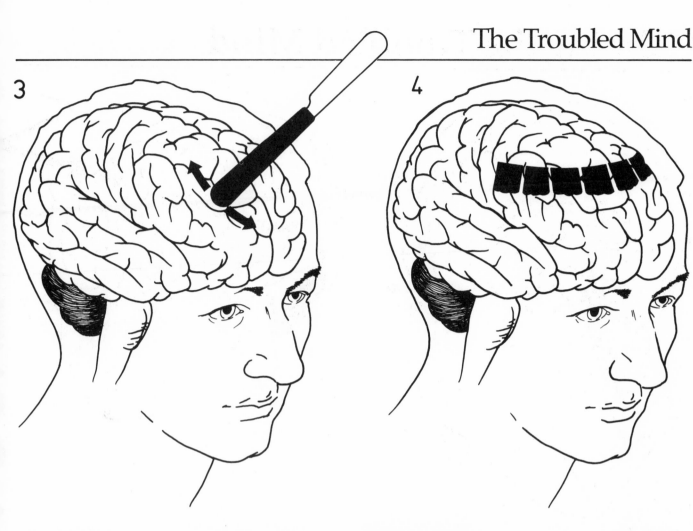

3 Frontal Lobotomy
Early overenthusiasm for neurosurgical techniques resulted in an 'epidemic' of frontal lobotomies which were often ill-considered and crudely performed. The operation aimed to sever the fibers connecting the frontal lobes to the limbic system or, in the crudest operations, merely to destroy areas of the lobes themselves. Most patients were sufferers from anxiety or obsessional neurosis or severe depression. Most doctors now feel that we know too little about the brain to indulge in such 'blind' surgical techniques.

4 Radioactive Implant
A more recent surgical technique involves the placing within the frontal lobes of radioactive 'seeds' with a short half-life. The seeds destroy a limited area of tissue with minimal effect on the rest of the brain. Like frontal lobotomy, this procedure aims to help those suffering from severe depression and neuroses, and is only used as a last resort when drugs and ECT have failed.

Where drugs fail or prove slow to take effect, some doctors favor ECT (electroconvulsive therapy), especially for treating patients with severe depressions. Each patient receives a muscle-relaxing drug and general anesthetic. Then electrodes applied to the scalp deliver an electric current. This sparks off electrical brain activity like that of an epileptic fit, but without big convulsive movements of the limbs. Moments later, the patient wakens. Six treatments spread over a few weeks may help to treat intense depressions with no more than brief memory disturbance. Just how this method works remains unclear.
Where drugs, ECT and psychotherapy cannot help depression or obsessional neurosis, doctors may seek the last resort of psychosurgery. Crude operations to sever fibers between frontal lobes and limbic system (seat of the emotions) left many patients human "vegetables." Modern methods include implanting slim, radioactive rods in the brain to destroy selected regions of the frontal lobes. This proves more successful. However, surgeons cannot yet explain exactly what it does inside the brain, and psychosurgery still carries risks that make this treatment controversial.

© DIAGRAM

Chapter 10

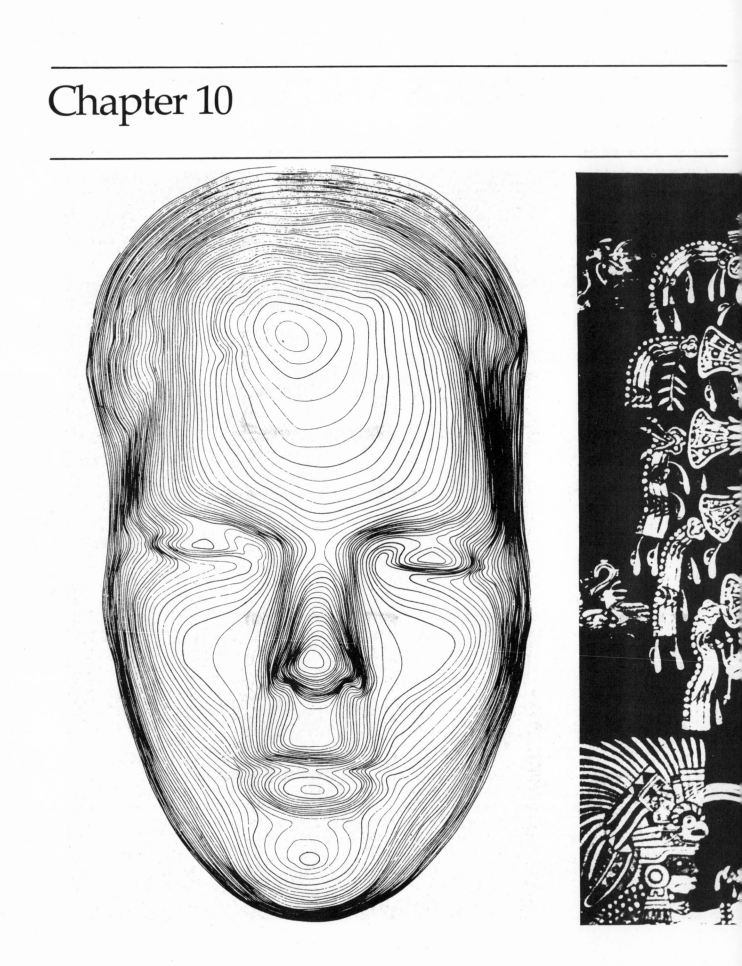

DRUGS AND DECEPTION

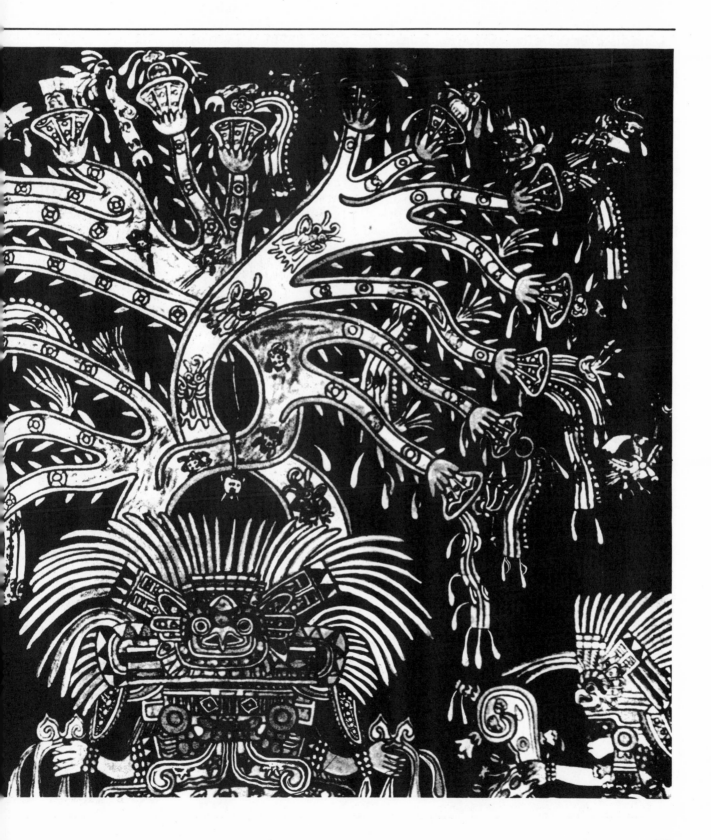

Painkillers

People have long known that certain drugs influence the brain, bringing sleep or stupor, or abnormal feelings of alertness and elation. New knowledge of brain chemistry is beginning to reveal just how these drugs cause their effects. Among the most amazing discoveries are those involving drugs that reduce sensitivity to pain.

Modern medicine employs an arsenal of painkilling agents. General anesthetics like chloroform and nitrous oxide (laughing gas) act on the brainstem to abolish consciousness. Local anesthetics like procaine deaden pain in a body area served by a sensory nerve; they act on the nerve membrane to block conduction through that nerve.

For otherwise unassailable discomforts such as headaches we use drugs that travel through the blood to all parts of the nervous system. The most widely used of these is acetylsalicylic acid, better known as aspirin – a substance originally found in willow bark, but now synthetically made. Aspirin evidently acts on pain centers in the thalamus deep inside the brain.

There are far more powerful analgesics (drugs subduing pain without removing consciousness). For severe, intractable pain doctors may prescribe heroin, morphine or another derivative of opium, a powder obtained from the seed-head of a poppy. Heroin and morphine bring relief from the severest pain and make even dying patients feel euphoric. Unhappily they prove addictive, and prolonged use may damage the brain and body.

To find safer alternatives scientists tried to discover how opiates suppress pain and why they are addictive. By the mid 1970s they had learned some answers, and much more besides. In short, American researchers found that opiates lock onto special receptor sites on nerve cell surfaces in the central nervous system. This slows down the rate at which those nerve cells fire off signals, and evidently that is what diminishes the sense of pain. Opiate receptors proved especially plentiful in the spinal cord, where most pain is initially processed, and opiates act strongly on the medial thalamus, the bit of brain giving awareness of deep, protracted pain.

The next intriguing discovery emerged in Scotland, where researchers identified a natural

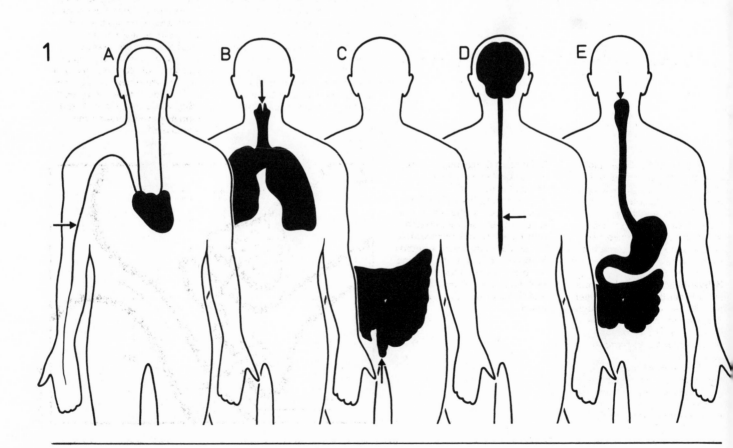

opiate which they named enkephalin ("in the head"). Enkephalin is a peptide – a short chain of those building blocks of protein the amino acids. Pain impulses entering the spinal cord make certain neurons yield enkephalins. These slot into other neurons' opiate receptors, blocking the release of neurotransmitters that would pass on the pain signal to the brain. Enkephalins located in the limbic system – the seat of the emotions – seemingly counteract depression, providing a natural equivalent of the euphoria induced by opium derivatives. Their addictive property can be explained by morphine's tendency to stop enkephalin output, so leaving receptor sites unfilled. The resulting pain is only eased by plugging the receptors with more morphine. Further research unmasked more natural opiates – this time in the pituitary gland. Named endorphins ("internal morphines") these are peptides too. Scientists now know of more than two dozen natural peptide neurotransmitters that help the body handle pain.

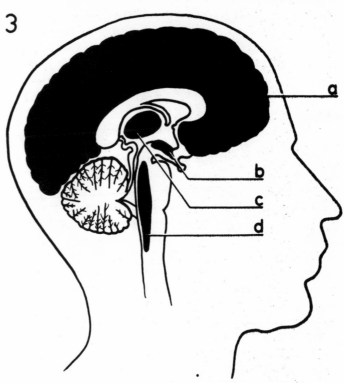

3

2

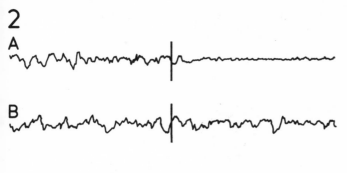

A

B

3 Areas of the Brain Affected
The cerebral cortex (**a**) is acted on by sedatives, while the hypothalamus (**b**) and thalamus (**c**) are noticeably affected by antidepressants and amphetamines. Many types of drug have an influence on the working of the reticular formation (**d**), either heightening consciousness (stimulants) or lowering it (sedatives and tranquilizers).

4 Enkephalins
The body's own painkillers are protein chains (**a**) fired from special nerve endings (**b**) into the receptor sites (**c**) of neurons transmitting pain signals (**d**). They inhibit the neuron producing neuro-transmitters that would pass on the signal, and so moderate the amount of pain we are aware of (**e**). Release of the enkephalins is triggered when neurons are stimulated by pain impulses entering the spinal cord.

1 How Drugs Enter the Body
Anesthetics, painkillers and drugs of all kinds can be taken in by a variety of routes.
A By injection into the bloodstream: drugs given by intravenous injection are very quickly distributed throughout the body by the pumping action of the heart.
B By inhalation – the thin lining of the lungs that absorbs oxygen into the blood also lets through drugs administered as gases.
C Via the rectum – the lining of the digestive tract absorbs drugs as it does food.
D Via the spinal cord (epidural): the drug enters the cerebrospinal fluid bathing the brain.
E By mouth – similar to **C**.

2 Effect of Drugs on the Brain
The EEGs (above) show the effect of a tranquilizer on electrical patterns within the brain. Trace **A** is the record of a rabbit's brain: before the bar a normal resting trace is recorded, but at that point a pain stimulus is applied, dramatically altering the brain wave. In trace **B** the rabbit has been given a drug, and the pain stimulus has little effect.

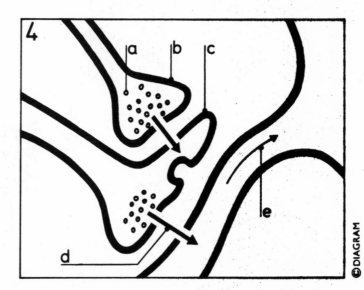

4

Depressants and Tranquilizers

Depressant drugs have a biochemical effect on the central nervous system; their actions on the brain make worried people feel sleepy or calmed. Different depressants have different effects. Narcotics like morphine also act as powerful (but addictive) painkillers (see pages 158–159). So-called hypnotic drugs act powerfully enough upon the brainstem's reticular activating system to bring sleep. These drugs include barbiturates like amytal and phenobarbitone. By about 1970 one writer calculated that such sleeping pills accounted for every tenth night's sleep in the United Kingdom. Unhappily, people become dependent on barbiturates. Habitual users who suddenly give up these pills suffer convulsions. Moreover, big barbiturate overdoses have caused deliberate and accidental suicides. Accordingly doctors have now switched their insomniac patients to safer drugs such as nitrazepam.

Alcohol is another powerful depressant, although people think of alcoholic drinks as stimulants. Like barbiturates, alcohol acts on the brain by boosting the activity of the neurotransmitter gamma amino butyric acid. Strong drink only seems to stimulate the brain, because its first effects are subduing the higher centers – those responsible for self-restraint and moral judgment. Freed from such inhibitions, lower regions of the brain gain the upper hand, so that mood and emotion rule the mind. If alcohol goes on accumulating in the blood it acts also on the lower centers of the brain, bringing slurred speech, unsteady gait, maybe unconsciousness, and possibly even death.

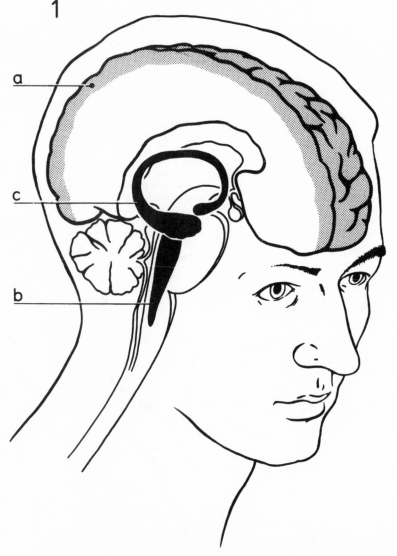

1 Areas Affected
Alcohol, a depressant, affects various parts and functions of the brain as its level builds up in the blood, but most depressant and tranquilizing drugs are quite specific in their mode of action. Hypnotics work powerfully on the cortex (**a**) and reticular formation (**b**), damping down electrical activity in the brain. Tranquilizers act on the reticular formation and limbic system (**c**), calming without causing sleep.

Normal   Depressant

2 Effects of Depressants
Pupil size (top right) may indicate use of depressants. The chart on the right shows the range of effects of each drug or group of drugs.

1 Depression.
2 Sedation.
3 Drowsiness.
4 Sleep.
5 Loss of pain.
6 Addiction.
7 Loss of sensation.
8 Convulsions.
9 Death.

A Tranquilizers (diazepam etc).
B Marijuana.
C Narcotics.
D Alcohol.
E Barbiturates.

Although alcoholism impairs the brain, its effects show up only slowly. One survey of 100 men after 17 years' daily consumption of 150 grams of alcohol (equivalent to 8 pints of beer or half a bottle of spirits) showed no obvious mental impairment. However, subtle tests of alcoholics with apparently normal brains prove them worse than other people at problem solving, abstract thought, memory and psychomotor speed. Brain scans show most alcoholics have shrunken brains – though arguably this is simply due to loss of fluid. Alcoholics turned abstainers are likely to regain at least some loss of brain weight and to improve their psychological performance.

Tranquilizers are calming drugs. Neuroleptics, or major tranquilizers, sedate without causing sleep. They include drugs like reserpine, which acts by reducing the brain's levels of chemical compounds called amines. Phenothiazines and butyrophenes have largely replaced reserpine, for they are freer from adverse side effects. The phenothiazine drug chlorpromazine usefully acts on the neurotransmitter dopamine, so helping to control schizophrenia and mania.

Anxiolytic sedatives, or minor tranquilizers, cannot cope with psychoses, but manage anxiety states. Chlordiazepoxide, diazepam and nitrazepam are among the best known such drugs. Most are safe, even taken in large doses. But drug-dependent people who stop taking these pills may suffer unpleasant withdrawal symptoms.

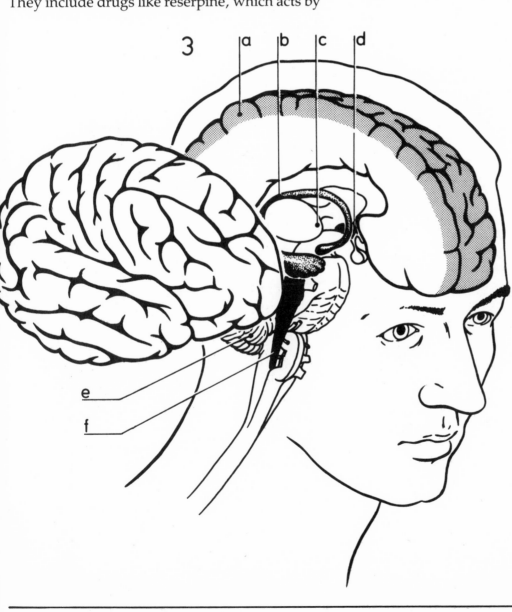

3 Alcohol and the Brain
The popular idea of alcohol acting as a stimulant is a complete – and dangerous – misunderstanding. It is a depressant, and its effect is accumulative. The reason for its apparently uninhibiting effect is that the higher centers of the brain's cortex (**a**), which control reasoning and judgment, are knocked out first. Mood centers like the limbic system (**b**), the thalamus (**c**) and the hypothalamus (**d**) are therefore allowed to run amok. Excess alcohol in the system affects the cerebellum (**e**) and the reticular formation (**f**), which control balance, coordination, consciousness and breathing.

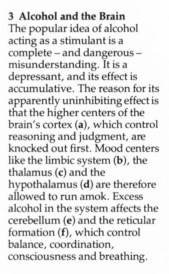

©DIAGRAM

Stimulants and Antidepressants

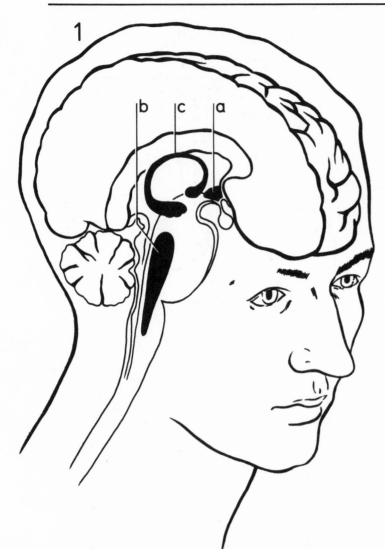

1 Areas of the Brain Affected
Stimulants act on the hypothalamus (**a**) and reticular formation (**b**), making the taker feel more alert by enhancing electrical activity within the brain. Antidepressants work on the limbic system (**c**) to control mood. Note the contrast between effects of depressants and tranquilizers (page 160), and those of stimulants and depressants, on reticular formation and limbic system.

2 Effects of Stimulants
Pupil size (lower right) may indicate use of stimulants. The chart on the right shows the range of effects of each drug or group of drugs. Contrast with the chart on page 160.

1 Stimulation.
2 Euphoria.
3 Palpitations.
4 Nervous tremors.
5 Convulsions.
6 Death.

A Hallucinogens.
B Marijuana.
C Antidepressants.
D Amphetamines.
E Strychnine.

Normal   Stimulants

While some drugs depress the central nervous system's activity, others stimulate it. Many people regularly smoke tobacco, which contains the stimulant nicotine. Most of us take mild stimulants every day in drinks like coffee, cocoa, tea and colas. Cocoa and tea respectively contain the stimulants theobromine and theophylline. All the drinks just mentioned contain caffeine – an even stronger stimulant. Acting on the brainstem's reticular formation – monitor of consciousness – the caffeine in one cup of coffee is enough to enliven the brain's flow of thoughts and output of motor signals to the muscles, and to make a tired and sleepy person more alert and wakeful. Too much caffeine brings insomnia, and ringing in the ears. It also speeds up heartbeat and respiration. Yet in fact few people suffer noticeable side effects. Caffeine's chemical structure resembles that of uric acid, found in the blood of man, apes and

monkeys, but destroyed by special enzymes in most other vertebrates. One theory suggests that uric acid thus acts like caffeine, providing a built-in nervous stimulant that helps explain the primates' high intelligence. Intriguingly, research indicates that a high uric acid level in the blood goes with qualities like drive and leadership.
Far more powerful stimulants than caffeine are the drugs amphetamine and cocaine. A synthetic product resembling ephedrine (obtained from a Chinese herb), amphetamine occurs as tablets, powder or in ampoules for injection. Chemically akin to that natural neurotransmitter noradrenalin, amphetamine enhances noradrenalin's activity within the brain by releasing quantities of this transmitter stored in nerve cells and preventing its reabsorption in the normal way. Possibly amphetamine also acts on the receptor areas of responsive target cells.

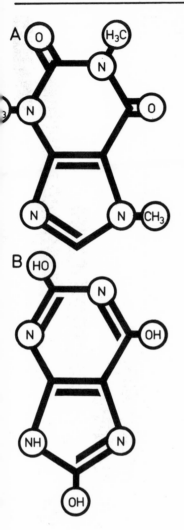

3 Caffeine and Uric Acid
Caffeine, a commonly used stimulant, has a chemical structure (**A**) that resembles that of uric acid (**B**), a substance found in the blood of man, apes and monkeys. In most animals, special enzymes break down uric acid, and it has been suggested that this natural stimulant is responsible for the higher intelligence of the primates. High uric acid levels in man have been associated with qualities of drive and leadership, but also, it should be mentioned, with gout!

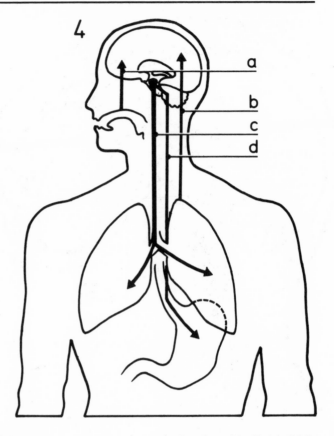

4 Nicotine
The stimulant drug nicotine is found in tobacco and has a range of effects upon the body (above). It is absorbed into the blood and then the brain through the mucous linings of the mouth (**a**) and lungs (**b**). Feedback through the nervous system (**c**) alters the width of the trachea, bronchi and alveoli (all types of airway leading to, and inside, the lungs). Nicotine circulating in the blood reaches the hypothalamus (**d**) and affects the appestats (hunger-monitoring mechanisms).

The effects upon the brain are quite dramatic. Individuals feel alert, elated; need less food and sleep; yet have improved athletic capability and capacity for performing simple mental tasks. Doctors accordingly once favored amphetamines to curb appetite in the obese, and to treat depression due to poor noradrenalin transmission between nerve cells. Students working overnight toward examinations, long-distance truck drivers, and athletes have all claimed benefits from taking amphetamine "uppers" or "pep pills." However, users found there was a price to pay in increased edginess, dry mouth, headache, palpitations, sweating, and possibly dependence on the drug with even worse after-effects including schizophrenia-like symptoms. One worldwide survey showed that from 8 to 10 per cent of people admitted to jails, psychiatric units and remand homes had been users of amphetamine.

Dependence on cocaine is just as dangerous. Addicts sniffing cocaine as a powder or injecting it beneath the skin are liable to suffer agitation, antisocial behavior, hallucinations and other kinds of serious mental disturbance.
Rather than rely riskily on drugs like these to counteract depression, doctors tend to use the safer so-called antidepressants. These control mood by acting on the midbrain and adjusting amine levels in the brain. Antidepressants take various forms: for instance vitamin B6 has been proved effective in counteracting female depression. The antidepressants known as MAOIs (monoamine oxidase inhibitors) can also be very useful, although unfortunately they react fatally with some foods, notably cheese.

©DIAGRAM

Hallucinogens

As their name suggests, hallucinogens are drugs that cause hallucinations by interfering with the normal balance of the brain. Mimicking certain naturally occurring chemical transmitters in the brain, these drugs affect the limbic system and nerves supplying the brainstem. People taking hallucinogens – especially the strongest types, termed psychedelics – feel intensely aware of all sensations and respond to quite ordinary sights or sounds with heightened emotion.

Hallucinogens come in four main groups, each containing drugs derived from plants. Harmatine, ibogaine, LSD (lysergic acid diethylamide) and psilocybin belong to the so-called indole alkaloid derivatives. Atropine, belladonna and scopolamine are all piperidine derivatives. Amphetamine and mescaline are two of the phenylethylamines. The fourth group consists of cannabinols, found in cannabis, a group of plants locally called marijuana, hashish, kif, etc.

LSD and most other hallucinogens stimulate the body's sympathetic nervous system, raising pulse rate and blood pressure, and producing sweating and palpitation. Hallucinogens chemically akin to noradrenalin and other agents that transmit signals through the central nervous system affect nerves linked to the reticular formation in the brainstem, overloading sensory pathways. This explains why individuals grow acutely conscious of what they feel, hear, see, taste and smell. Involvement of the limbic system adds an emotional dimension to this effect. Meanwhile hallucinogens suppress brain centers controlling judgment, memory, and feelings, so that the individual behaves more like child than adult. Hallucinations are usually visual, from flashes of light to complex scenes.

Effects on any individual depend partly on the type of drug. Some drugs promote fantasy, others, feelings. Thus research suggests that harmaline sparks off vivid imagery while MDA (methyl-dioxy-amphetamine) boosts the taker's ego. Impact is also influenced by size of dose. Small doses may produce no more than extra-clear consciousness. Large doses of LSD made the French artist Henri Michaux sense that he was floating in his body, painfully aware of trivial sensations, expecting objects to become alive, and aware that ordinary people seemed beneficent or sinister.

Personality and circumstances play a part. Novices may suffer nausea, anxiety, depression. For experienced users, onset of an experience may bring euphoria, pleasant tingling and irrational thoughts that seem enormously significant. Some users' out-of-body or other mystical experiences have led them to mistake the brain's disorganized behavior for an elevated state of consciousness. Some users high on psychedelic drugs have even leaped fatally from tall buildings convinced that they could fly. Other risks may possibly arise in sharp mood swings from mania to deep depression, induced by large doses. Hallucinogens are not normally addictive, though susceptible individuals can become dependent on them. They have some use in psychotherapy.

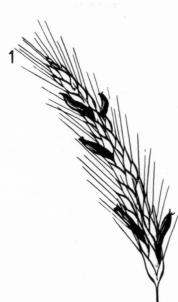

1 Indole Alkaloid Derivatives
LSD (lysergic acid diethylamide) is an example of the harmine group of hallucinogens. It is derived from a poisonous fungus, ergot, which grows on rye and used to cause widespread outbreaks of poisoning (ergotism) when infected kernels were milled and made into bread.

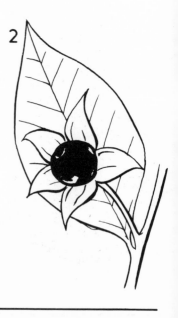

2 Piperidine Derivatives
Atropa belladonna (deadly nightshade) contains several psychoactive alkaloids including hyoscyamine and scopolamine. The plant itself is poisonous and is believed to have been used in witches' brews, but substances derived from it have important uses in modern medicine.

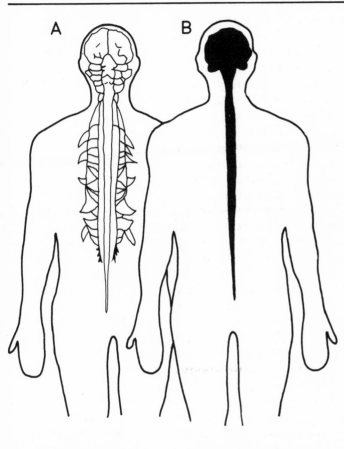

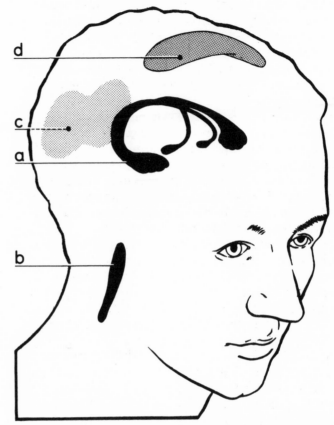

How Hallucinogens Work

LSD and most other hallucinogens stimulate the sympathetic nervous system, shown above (**A**). This results in a rise in pulse rate and blood pressure, and produces sweating and palpitations. Cannabinols, however, may have a calming effect, reducing stomach acid secretion. Some hallucinogens act like noradrenalin and other agents that transmit nerve messages within the central nervous system, shown above (**B**). These drugs cause overloading of sensory pathways, making the user very conscious of all sensation.

Areas of the Brain Affected

Hallucinogens have strong effects on the limbic system (**a**), influencing mood and emotions, and on the reticular formation (**b**), making the user acutely conscious of sensory input. Visual centers (**c**) react by producing visions, ranging from flashes of light to complex scenes. Memory centers (**d**) are suppressed, together with other higher cerebral functions such as judgment. The combination of effects on the limbic system, such as violent mood swings and loss of judgment, may prove dangerous to the user of these drugs.

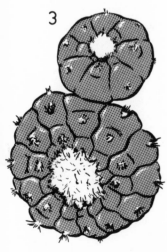

3 Phenylethylamines

The cactus shown has been known for hundreds of years as a hallucinogen by Mexican Indians, to whom the mescal or peyote button has an important religious significance. The buttons, which are cut from the cactus and dried, contain psychoactive alkaloids inducing colorful visions when taken.

4 Cannabinols

Cannabis sativa is widely grown throughout the world, being known in different areas by various names, according to whether the dried plant or the resin it exudes under hot conditions are being referred to. Cannabis is usually smoked or eaten, and produces a feeling of relaxation and cheerfulness.

©DIAGRAM

Manipulating the Mind

This chapter has already shown that drugs can tamper with the brain. Unscrupulous authorities can – some do – employ drugs and other means to manipulate the mind.

War and crime movies familiarize us with notions of using drugs to worm secrets from unwilling captives or alter an individual's behavior. In fact so-called truth drugs like sodium thiopentone are less effective than you might expect. They simply make people drowsy, acting much like alcohol by lowering the brain's inhibitory guards. Research with animals suggests the possibility of improving or destroying memory, although attempts to test magnesium pemoline as an old person's memory enhancer have failed.

Other experiments on animals suggest remote possibilities of transforming normal individuals into pacifists or killers respectively by feeding carbachol or atropine to a key region of the brain. Theoretically a dictator could pacify an entire nation just by adding tranquilizers to the public water supply. For wartime use, the hallucinogenic agent code-named BZ, delivered as an aerosol spray, could make the enemy confused, giddy, disoriented, hallucinated and liable to outbursts of maniacal behavior.

Far more frightful are the deadly nerve gases which flood the nervous system with acetylcholine so that victims cannot operate any muscles and soon die from asphyxiation.

Fortunately for our peace of mind, the mass use of mind-bending or nerve-disrupting drugs is unlikely to escape the realm of fantasy, if only because effective distribution cannot be assured. Even using drugs to brainwash individuals does not always work, for susceptibility to particular

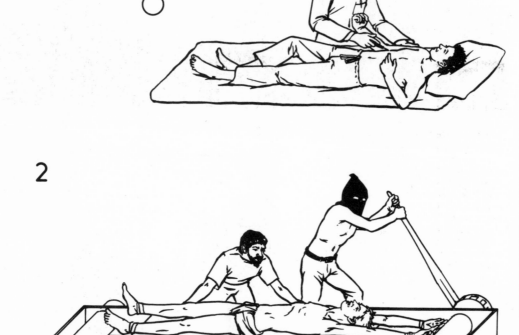

1 Truth Drugs
Drugs such as sodium pentothal, the molecular structure of which is shown (far left), were thought at first to have great potential for gaining confessions from spies and criminals. This early enthusiasm proved unfounded as we now know that it is quite possible for someone to keep telling a lie when under the influence of such a drug. But these substances have proved useful in psychiatry as they lower the brain's inhibitory guards, helping patients recall experiences and emotions they had tried to suppress.

2 Brainwashing
Drugs are not a reliable way of manipulating the brain, as other factors such as personality and physical endurance are involved. A person who is capable of resisting suggestion of physical torment may succumb to isolation and feelings of being alone. Medieval torture chambers, with their dank, dismal surroundings and the unlikelihood of escape, were probably as effective in their purpose as any truth drug.

drugs varies from person to person.
Drugs, though, are not the only route into a person's mind. Isolation can powerfully disturb the brain, making some individuals increasingly suggestible to propaganda, as Chinese interrogators proved with some American captives in the Korean War. Intrigued by this technique, and curious to learn how lonely occupations can affect the mind, Montreal's McGill University in 1951 launched sensory-deprivation experiments with volunteers as human guinea pigs. In some such tests, subjects lie quietly alone for hours or days in darkened, soundproof cubicles, wearing gloves and earplugs. One-third give up early. Many of the rest show slowed alpha brain waves, suffer delusions, and reveal temporarily impaired mental functioning. Subjects respond well to questions calling for specific answers, but perform poorly in creativity tests. Ability to perceive color, recognize shapes by feeling them, and coordinate the body's muscles all decline. Also beliefs and attitudes may prove readily remolded.

Sensory deprivation and closely allied perceptual-deprivation experiments especially affect the brainstem's reticular formation, a key structure in the processes involved in attention, perception and motivation.

Plainly, then, for full efficiency, the brain depends upon a steady flow of information about its surroundings. This has implications for the bedridden, jail-bound, and those performing boring or lonely work, especially in small rooms lacking windows with an outside view.

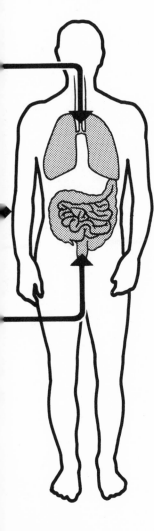

3 Nerve Gases
These deadly substances may enter the body in three ways. Gas may be inhaled through mouth and nose (**A**), or taken in on contaminated food. Liquid gas landing on the skin (**B**), particularly on a wound, is absorbed into the body. Gas can also enter the body through the excretory exits (**C**).

4 Nerve Toxins
Even the tiniest dose of one nerve toxin, Botulin X or A, is capable of paralyzing the nervous system and causing death. If one gram (the weight of a baked bean) of this substance was applied to the skin wounds of 14,285,714 people, half of them would be affected – roughly the entire population of New York City.

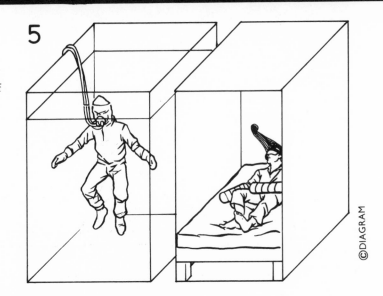

5 Sensory Deprivation
Experiments which isolate individuals from any kind of sensory input (as far as that is possible) show that the brain relies upon a continuous flow of information for proper functioning. Without stimulation, subjects begin to hallucinate and their ability to perform simple tasks is temporarily impaired.

©DIAGRAM

Chapter 11

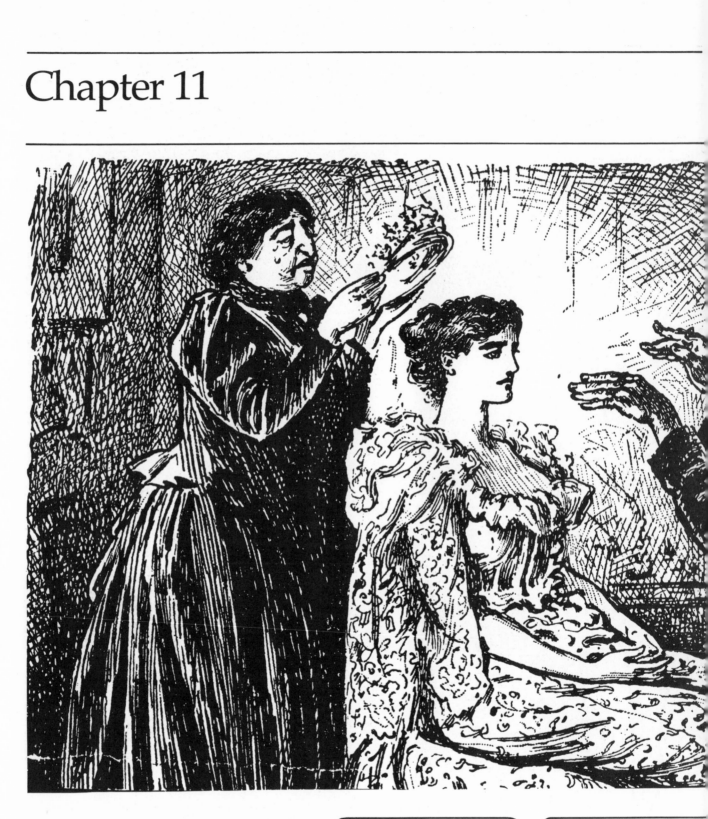

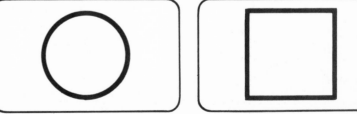

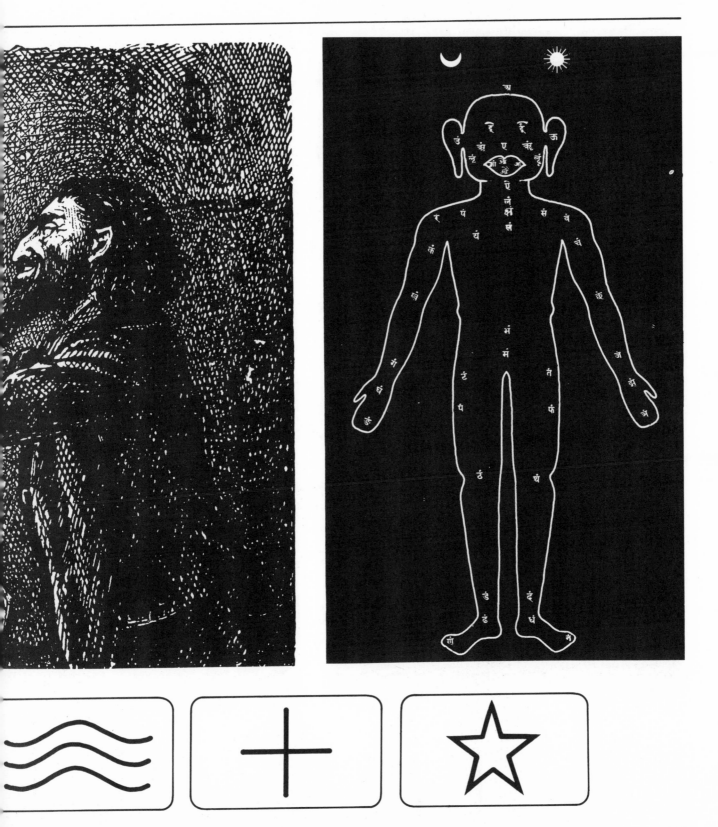

Hypnosis

Doctors busily discarding superstition once ridiculed claims that the mind produced effects defying scientific explanation. Hypnosis, yoga, extrasensory perception – phenomena like these still largely baffle us, but now scientists at least concede they merit serious attention.

People had unknowingly practiced hypnotism for centuries before Franz Anton Mesmer made his first experiments in 1776. Misconceived by him as "animal magnetism" and later misnamed from the Greek *hypnos* ("sleep"), hypnotism has been described more fittingly as "a temporary condition of altered attention induced by another person." Someone being fully hypnotized passes through three main stages: light, medium and deep trance. Only the most suggestible of people – about 1 in 20

– can be deeply hypnotized. Unwilling subjects remain quite unaffected. The usual hypnotizing process involves the subject lying or sitting comfortably relaxed while gazing at a shiny object and listening to the hypnotist's voice monotonously repeating suggestions that induce hypnosis. The main point is to shut out all stimuli but those tending to send the subject into hypnotic trance. This can also be accomplished in other ways, for instance, by hearing one's own pre-recorded breathing played back amplified, or by gazing at light shone through revolving prisms. Hypnotized people have a glazed, humorless, withdrawn appearance, yet may behave quite normally unless the hypnotist suggests differently. Then astonishing results may follow.

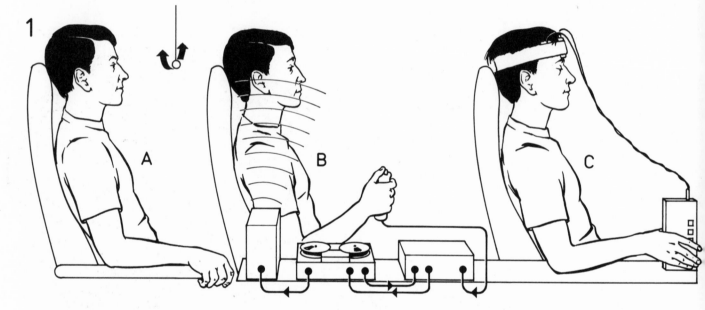

1 How Hypnotism is Induced
Most people are hypnotized by a hypnotist using the standard techniques of a bright swinging object together with suggestions repeated in a monotonous voice (**A**). The subject must be comfortable and relaxed and, above all, open to suggestion. It is impossible to hypnotize an unwilling subject.

Self-hypnosis is also possible. The hypnotist's voice may be recorded on tape and played back by the subject. After each suggestion, the subject presses a remote control device to go on to the next stage (**B**). This puts control of the procedure in the hands of the subject and shows that hypnosis is a more simple technique than many practitioners of method A might admit.

It is possible to induce sleep in insomniacs simply by using a device which sends a low-frequency current through the brain, affecting sleep control centers (**C**). Similar electrical input devices may affect brain waves to produce hypnotic states.

On command, a hypnotized individual may lie rigidly across the backs of chairs while someone stands upon his body. Afterward, the subject may not remember anything of what has happened. In fact he may go on obeying some instruction received while hypnotized. This is known as post-hypnotic suggestion.

Skeptics claim that unhypnotized people can remain rigid, withstand pain and mimic other effects supposedly produced by trance conditions. Yet hypnosis does seem to have remarkable effects that cast new light on mind – body interaction. Thus touching a subject's skin with a pencil may produce blisters if he has been told the pencil is red hot. Touching a hypnotized subject's skin with a Japanese wax-plant failed to produce an expected skin reaction when the subject had been told it was a harmless chestnut leaf. Yet a chestnut leaf produced a weal when the subject thought it was a wax-plant leaf. Telling a subject to imagine he has just eaten a large, fatty meal stimulates his body to secrete lipase – a fat-digesting enzyme. When he thinks the meal was rich in protein, he manufactures pepsin and trypsin – protein-digesting enzymes. Hypnosis also can affect breathing, heart rate, and various kinds of glandular activity. The intriguing aspect of many of these tests is their effects upon body functions that had been long supposed to operate outside the mind's control – the same kind of phenomenon as noted in conditioned reflexes.

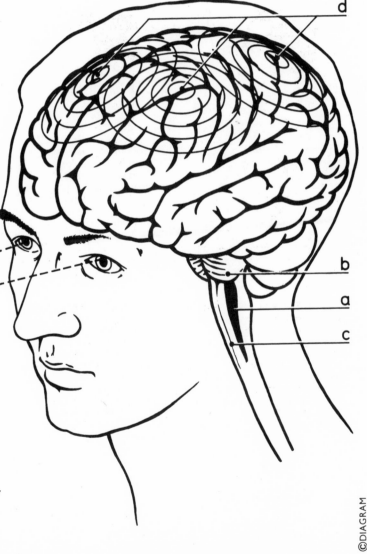

2 How Hypnotism Works
There are many theories on the exact effect hypnotism has on the brain's functioning. One of the most plausible theories is as follows.

When we concentrate our attention on a swinging ball, messages received through the eyes are relayed by visual pathway to the midbrain. Areas of the brain affected include the reticular formation (**a**), pons (**b**) and medulla (**c**), but the incoming messages primarily influence and inhibit the midbrain centers, so that the responses of the motor and sensory areas, and memory areas of the cerebrum (**d**) are influenced and modified. The effects of hypnosis are demonstrated by brain wave traces; **A** (above) is a normal trace with a characteristic spiky waveform, whereas **B**, taken from a hypnotized subject, shows increased amplification and reduced frequency.

©DIAGRAM

Yoga and Biofeedback

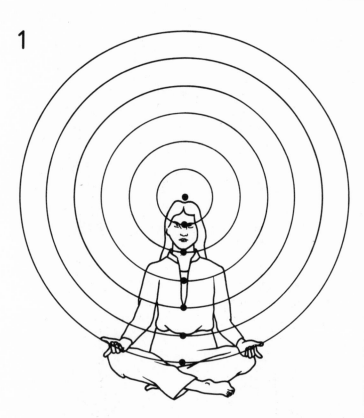

In India in 1970, television cameras filmed an almost unbelievable experiment. They recorded a man surviving for more than five hours in a sealed box where any ordinary person would have suffocated in that time. This man was special, though. Forty-six-year-old Ramanand Yogi was a Hindu who practiced *yoga* ("union") – a physical and mental discipline originally designed to unite man with Brahman, the World Soul. Instruments monitoring Ramanand Yogi's breathing in the box showed that he used little more than half the calculated minimum amount of oxygen required to keep himself alive. Indeed, for one hour he survived on a bare quarter of what his body should have needed.

In other tests, one yogi produced sweat on his forehead only. Another slowed down his heart rate while just sitting still. Yet others are known to lie at ease on beds of nails. Such mystics achieve what theories of brain function once held to be impossible: they are able to bring automatic body mechanisms under mind control. The secret of their skill seems to lie in the trance-like state induced by practicing techniques of meditation. Before experiments like Ramanand's proved man could master his own automatic body functions, American psychologist Neal Miller had shown that this was so for rats and dogs. By offering two batches of dogs the same reward for opposite responses, Miller conditioned one group to salivate more, the other, less. Tests with rats suggested that these could mentally control blood pressure, heart rate, intestinal contractions, and rate of urine formation. Moreover Miller showed their autonomic nervous systems could work selectively, not just affecting a whole group of bodily activities.

1 The Seven Chakras
According to Hindu philosophy, the cosmos consists of seven ascending planes, each of which has a focus in the body for the purposes of meditation. Each chakra or wheel is possessed of a different kind of energy, which can be interiorized through meditation. The mental and physical discipline of yoga is designed to unite man with Brahman at the highest level.

2 Physical Effects of Yoga
Claims that yogis could stop their hearts beating and survive being buried alive were tested by Indian scientists in the late 1960s. In one remarkable experiment, filmed in 1970, Ramanand Yogi was sealed in an airtight metal box (right). As he went into a trance, air samples measuring his body's uptake of oxygen were taken every half hour (far right). The yogi's usual rate of oxygen consumption (metabolic rate) is given for comparison. This experiment showed dramatically that yogis were indeed capable of slowing normal body processes.

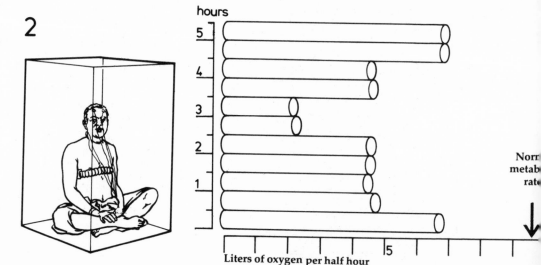

hours

Normal metabolic rate

Liters of oxygen per half hour

Such discoveries have convinced some doctors that we might help our bodies resist or even overcome disease by mind control techniques. Under names like biofeedback and autogenic training such methods are already showing promise. As with Eastern mystics, subjects cultivate a relaxed mental state by passive concentration. Many try imagining a pleasant situation, like strolling through a flowery meadow. Unlike yogis they are wired to electronic devices with lights, tones, or moving meter needles to feed back data on their own involuntary bodily activities, notably blood pressure and "brain waves." Properly relaxed patients can often influence these things. Several conditions seem especially well suited to biofeedback treatment. Victims of certain neuromuscular disorders may recover limb function by learning to reroute nerve signals to affected muscles. Migraine sufferers alter congested blood vessels near the brain by diverting extra blood into the hands. Epileptics suffer fewer fits and insomniacs sleep better if both learn to modify the brain's electrical activity. Even some allergies may benefit from biofeedback.
Similar mind control perhaps explains why rare people condemned to die from cancer literally seem to will their own recovery.
Biofeedback has limitations, but its potential may be largely still untapped.

4

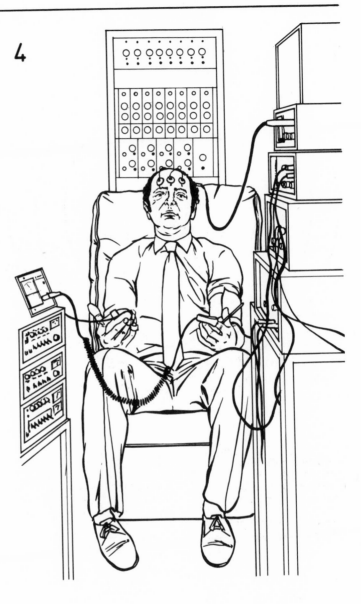

3

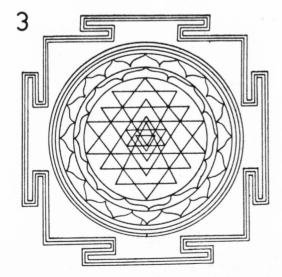

3 The Mandala
Designs such as the example illustrated are used as aids to meditation and have a spiritual significance as they represent an ordering of the universe and a focus for its forces. Drawings with a similar emphasis on square border and round central element are found in other cultures, and the psychologist Carl Jung attached special importance to mandalas drawn by patients. He felt that they represented attempts to reconcile the conscious with the subconscious mind.

4 Biofeedback
The man shown above is attempting to alter the way his body normally works by concentrating on the readings given by various instruments measuring brain waves, blood pressure, etc. This kind of relaxation technique, like yoga, has proved that the autonomic nervous system can, to some extent, be brought under conscious control. Biofeedback has already shown useful results in the treatment of certain disorders, such as epilepsy and migraine.

©DIAGRAM

The Brain and Beyond

So far in this book we have been considering the brain as a machine whose output depends essentially on input fed in through the senses. Yet history is rich in anecdotes of individuals whose minds seemed capable of more: people claiming knowledge that their brains could not have gained through any of the senses known to science. Since serious-minded men founded the Society for Psychical Research in London a century ago, scientists have run thousands of experiments to learn if minds indeed have supernormal powers. Most tests investigated one or other of three main "faculties": telepathy, clairvoyance and precognition, collectively called extrasensory perception by American psychologist J.B. Rhine. Dating from the early 1930s, Rhine's tests at Duke University in Durham, North Carolina, remain the most quoted examples of an experimental blitzkrieg on problems of parapsychology. Many of these tests involved identifying unseen cards from a 25-card Zener deck. This deck contains five types of card, each featuring a different symbol. Thus random guessing should produce a success rate of only 1 in 5.

To test telepathy (thought transference) Rhine had one person think of symbols in a random order while another tried to name the sequence. In a general extrasensory (ESP) test the sender gazed at each card in turn.

Clairvoyance (knowledge of information not necessarily known to anyone by ordinary means) was tested for by having subjects name the card sequence in a shuffled deck of face-down cards.

To probe precognition (supernormal knowledge of future events) subjects named each card in a mechanically shuffled deck seconds before that card was shown. Predicting the throw of dice was another precognition test employed.

Three years of Rhine's telepathy and clairvoyance testing averaged 7 successes out of every 25, 2 better than chance would have produced, an overall result millions to one against the odds. Interestingly, success rates tended to peak early in a session, tail off, then pick up again. Extrasensory perception appeared to be only a weak, unconscious, uncontrollable and unreliable faculty. Skeptics criticizing Rhine's procedure even doubted that ESP was proven. Yet many scientists believe there must be "something there" – perhaps the same something that makes some people claim they know when they are being watched, or leap aside instinctively from sudden unseen danger (though both can be explained in other ways). Under scientifically controlled conditions, few people claiming ESP or similar abilities have been able to convince scientists of their authenticity.

Just what that something is remains debatable. One neurobiologist sees the brain detecting influences from the mind, considered as distinct and yet intangible. Others suggest the brain can send and receive invisible electromagnetic waves like those beaming radio and television signals to our homes. Such explanations scarcely cover precognition or clairvoyance. Maybe we yet know little more about the full capacity of brain power than eighteenth-century scientists understood of magnetism and electricity.

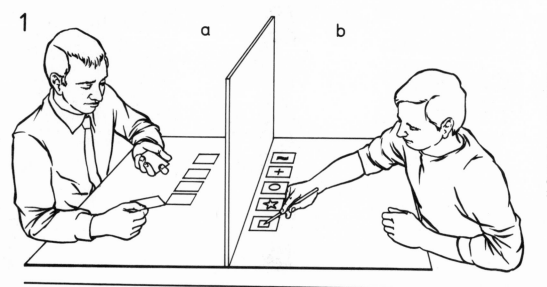

1 Testing for ESP
In this test, the sender (a) is noting the symbol on each card turned up from a shuffled pack, and attempting to transmit this information by extrasensory perception to the receiver (b). The receiver points to the card that he thinks matches the card turned up by the sender. Rhine's results in these tests over three years achieved a success rate of 7 in 25, instead of the 5 in 25 that would be expected if the receiver were merely guessing.

Now we know that brain power can control normally automatic body processes, thought transference and maybe even precognition seem slightly less impossible. But what of the mind's role in apparently creating matter or moving it around? Some researchers believe that such things as apparitions and poltergeists (mischievous spirits) are no less products of the mind than ordinary reasoning – it's just that so far we have not found how the appropriate mental mechanisms work.

Undeterred by lack of evidence, theorists have come up with many explanations. According to one still influential theory dating from the 1880s, apparitions are often telepathic signals sent by an individual at a time of crisis to a person who perceives the message as if it reached the brain through the ordinary senses. If the percipient in turn transmits what he perceives, others near him see the apparition, too. If this is true, such "objective" apparitions differ from subjective hallucinations which of course are just internal products of an individual's disordered brain. Arguably, apparitions of the dead then become "delayed" telepathic signals transmitted by people just about to die or – if you believe the mind is not a product of the brain – signals projected from minds surviving after death.

Better documented than most apparitions, yet less readily explained, are so-called poltergeist activities. These typically involve rapping, shifting furniture, or throwing plates, knives or groceries around. Recorded incidents date from the Dark Ages. Many proved no more than frauds. But even skeptical parapsychologists had no easy explanation for the bottles they saw sliding off a table at one Long Island house in 1958, and there are other well authenticated instances. Interestingly, most happen in homes containing psychologically disturbed girls around the age of puberty. This suggests some people can move objects by mind power alone. Shifted objects have included cupboards too heavy for any ordinary child to budge.

Scientific tests for psychokinesis (moving things by mind power) have had more modest aims, like willing dice to fall a certain way. The first tests failed to take into account such factors as bias produced by the hollowing out of spots on dice so that the "one" side is slightly heavier than the "six" side. Then, too, even adjusted tests carried out by different groups produced conflicting findings. Psychokinesis remains unproven, but with large parts of the brain yet unmapped, who knows just what its limits are?

Even without invoking supernature, the future for the brain appears sufficiently intriguing – especially in functional research and medicine. Already microelectrodes implanted in the brain and hitched up to computers or portable devices have moved limbs for people paralyzed by strokes, controlled epileptic seizures, and relieved chronic pain. Soon, portable vision prostheses may provide blind people with some sort of sight. Experiments with Rhesus monkeys suggest that even brain transplants are technically possible. Technology can help to mend the brain. It can even mimic some kinds of brain activity. Yet for subtle complexity no conceivable computer can match the mechanism lodged inside your skull.

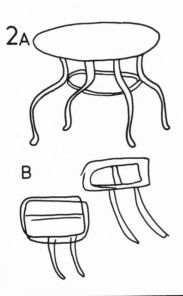

2 Drawing by Telepathy
Some tests for telepathy have taken the form of the sender doing a fairly detailed drawing and the receiver attempting to reproduce the drawing through information relayed telepathically. The table (**A**) drawn by the sender resulted in the two smaller drawings (**B**) from the receiver.

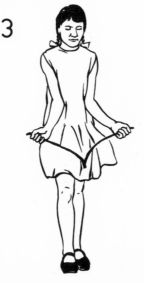

3 Dowsing
Dowsing, or water-divining, is a very ancient art, and involves finding water under the ground when none is obvious from physical signs. The dowser holds the two ends of a divining rod (usually made of hazel) as shown, and walks slowly over the ground until the rod dips sharply in response to some outside influence.

© DIAGRAM

Chapter 12

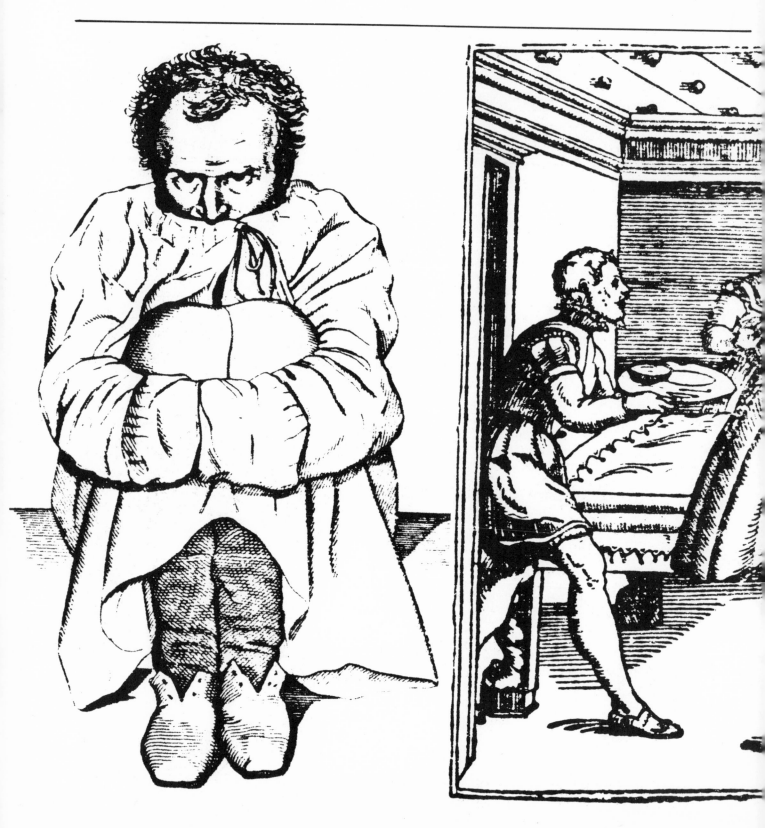

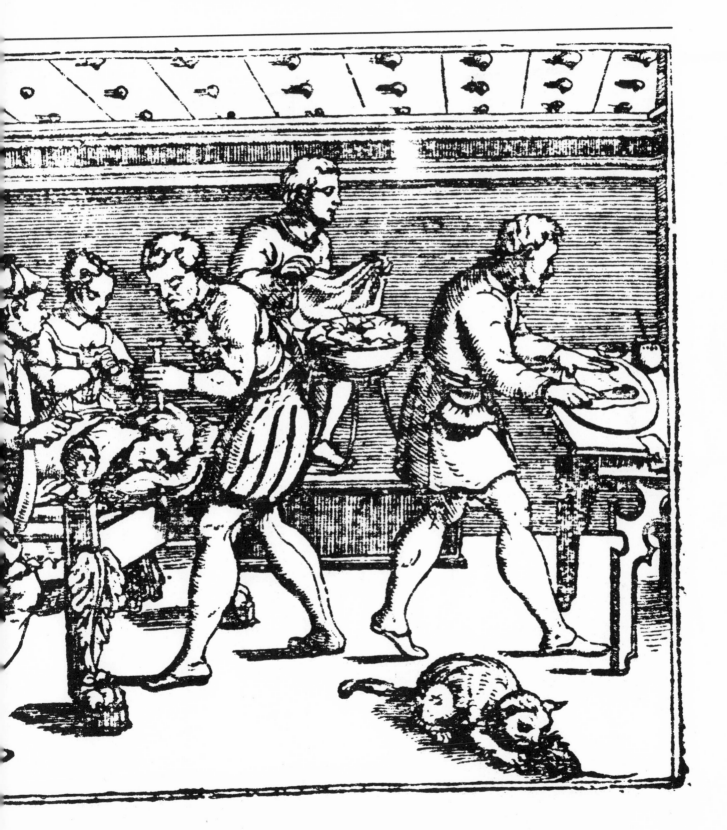

Landmarks in Research: 1

The following eight pages provide a broadly chronological illustrated survey of the major milestones in man's efforts to map, explore and understand the human brain. By necessity it is highly selective – the first few pages taking us from the ancient Greeks to the close of the eighteenth century, while the next few pages cover the surge of scientific enquiry that took place in the nineteenth century. The pages relating to the present century, though highly condensed, are still barely able to do justice to the hundreds of physicians, psychiatrists and psychologists throughout the world who today are working hand in hand with researchers from every other branch of science and technology to unravel the complexities of the human mind.

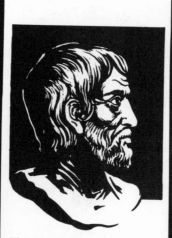

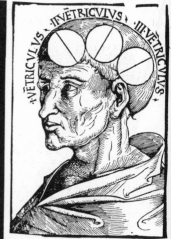

The Greek philosopher Pythagoras (6th century BC) suggested that the brain was the organ of the mind.

Herophilus of Chalcedon (about 300 BC) saw the brain as the central part of the nervous system. He rightly associated nerves with movement and sensation.

Eristratus of Chios (after 300 BC) described the brain's main parts, also meninges and ventricles. He guessed that brain convolutions held a key to human intelligence.

Aretaeus of Cappadocia (AD 81–?138) distinguished between mental and nervous diseases and described aspects of epilepsy.

Soranus of Ephesus (AD 98–138) began classifying mental diseases and laid down humane treatments for them.

Medieval thinkers held that sensory analysis, reason, and memory inhabited three linked brain cavities or ventricles.

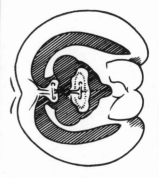

About 1505 Leonardo da Vinci made the first wax cast of brain ventricles (an ox's). He shifted the supposed site of sensory analysis (*sensus communis*) to the second ventricle, formerly the supposed seat of reason – hence, maybe, our current use of the term "commonsense."

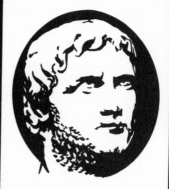

The Greek physician Galen (2nd century AD) established garbled theories of the brain and other parts of the body that prevailed for 1500 years.

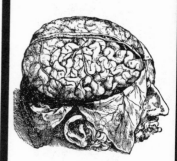

Andreas Vesalius of Brussels in 1543 produced the first "modern" anatomy of the brain, based on detailed drawings of corpses. Vesalius debunked the medieval notion that the ventricles housed separate mental faculties.

The Rhineland physician Johan Wyer (1515–88) showed that witches were just people with mental afflictions.

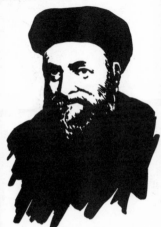

Italian anatomist Gabriele Fallopio incompletely described the cranial nerves in 1561.

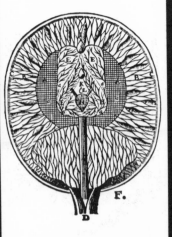

René Descartes, French founder of modern philosophy, in 1637 divorced soul from brain. His theory underpinned a belief that mind is not a mere product of the brain.

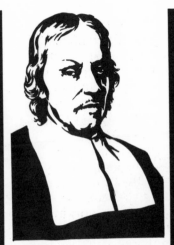

Italian anatomist and pioneer microscopist Marcello Malpighi (1628–94) studied brain cells by microscope.

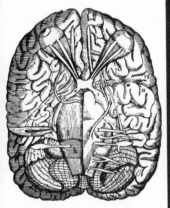

The Italian Constanzo Varoli illustrated the pons (1573), part of the brainstem that Vesalius had missed.

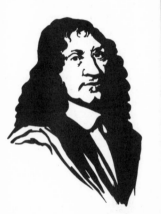

Dutch professor Franz de le Boe (1614–72), known as Franciscus Sylvius, gave his name to the fissure of Sylvius – a great groove in each side of the cerebral cortex.

Johann Jakob Wepfer of Basel in 1658 declared that burst blood vessels in the brain caused apoplexy (strokes).

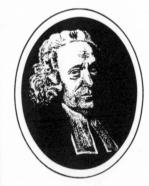

The English physiologist Stephen Hales discovered about 1730 that reflex movements in a frog's legs depended upon the spinal cord.

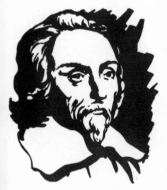

William Harvey (1578–1657), English discoverer of the circulation of the blood, thought sensory nerves took sensations to the brain, and motor nerves worked muscles.

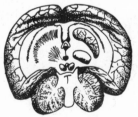

Thomas Willis of Oxford (1621–75) gave an improved account of cranial nerves. He traced blood flow to the brain and held that thought took place in its big, wrinkled cerebrum.

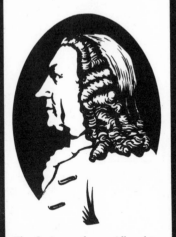

The Swiss professor Albrecht von Haller (1708–77) showed that feeling depends on nerves and nerves activate muscles. He traced nerves from limbs to cerebral cortex.

©DIAGRAM

Landmarks in Research: 2

The Neapolitan anatomist Domenico Cotugno in 1774 found that cerebrospinal fluid (not "animal spirit" as long supposed) filled the brain's cavities.

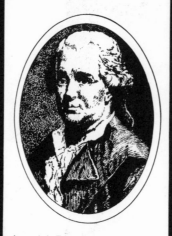

Austria's Franz Anton Mesmer (1734–1815) pioneered the use of hypnosis, known then as mesmerism.

French royal physician Félix Vicq d'Azyr (1748–1794) noted layers in a pickled brain cortex.

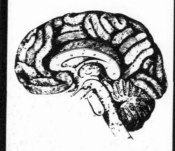

Italian anatomist Luigi Galvani (1737–98) showed that an electrical charge made muscles contract.

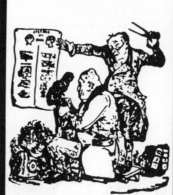

German physician Franz Joseph Gall (1758–1828) dissected the brain, so laying a basis for modern neurology. He co-founded phrenology.

Philippe Pinel, a Parisian physician, freed chained lunatics in 1793 and helped pioneer humane treatment for victims of mental disease.

Gaspard Vieusseux of Geneva gave the first clear account of cerebrospinal fever, 1806.

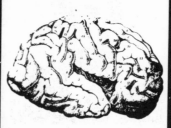

Sardinia's Luigi Rolando in 1809 declared the cerebrum handles deliberate acts, the cerebellum involuntary ones.

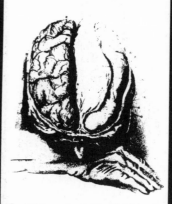

Scottish surgeon Sir Charles Bell in 1811 declared each nerve carries motor or sensory stimuli, not both.

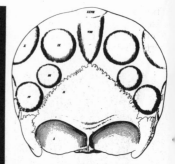

German physician Johann Kaspar Spurzheim (1776–1832) with Franz Gall developed phrenology, a pseudo science of reading character from "bumps" found on the head.

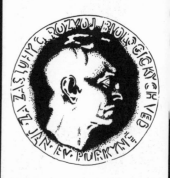

Czech physiologist Johannes Evangelista Purkinje in 1837 described the cerebellum's large "Purkinje" cells.

German physiologist Robert Remak in 1838 named the neurolemma (the myelin sheath around many nerve fibers).

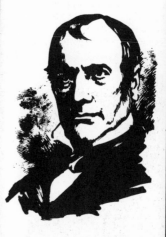

French physiologist Pierre Flourens (1794–1867) proved the brain's respiratory center lies low in the brainstem. He pioneered the idea of nervous coordination.

The first textbook of nervous diseases, by Moritz Heinrich Romberg of Berlin, appeared in parts, 1840–46.

Bartolomeo Panizza in 1855 proved parts of the cerebral cortex vital for vision.

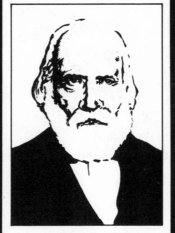

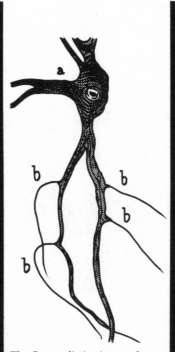

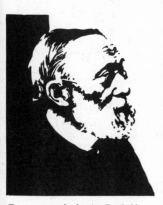

William T.G. Morton pioneered the use of general anesthesia for surgery at Boston, USA, in 1846.

British physiologist and neurologist Charles Édouard Brown-Séquard (1817–94) made major discoveries involving spinal cord and endocrine glands, and foreshadowed the discovery of neurotransmitters.

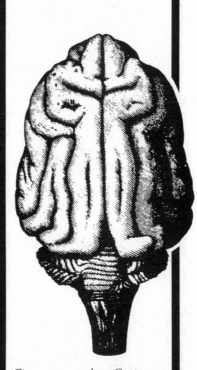

The first realistic picture of a neuron (by Otto Dieters of Bonn) was published in 1865.

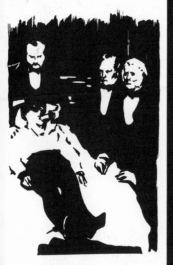

German physicist Hermann Ludwig Ferdinand von Helmholtz in 1852 measured the speed of nerve impulse (in a frog).

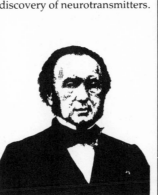

French physiologist Claude Bernard (1813–78) showed that the nervous system can control blood flow in the body.

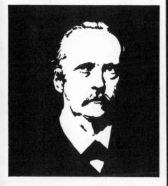

German pathologist Rudolf Virchow in 1854 named the neuroglia or supportive "glue cells" in the brain.

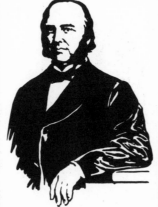

French surgeon Paul Broca in 1861 claimed that articulate speech depended on a site in the left cerebral hemisphere.

German researchers Gustav Theodor Fritsch and Eduard Hitzig in 1870 found that electric shocks to one of a dog's cerebral hemispheres produced movement of the other side of its body.

©DIAGRAM

Landmarks in Research: 3

German biochemist Johan Ludwig Wilhelm Thudichum pioneered the study of brain chemistry about 1870.

Italian physician Camillo Golgi in 1873 described a way of staining nerve cells to make them show up under the microscope.

German neurologist Carl Wernicke in 1874 discovered the brain area concerned with understanding words.

Wilhelm Heinrich Erb and Carl Friedrich Otto Westphal of Germany described the knee-jerk reflex in 1875.

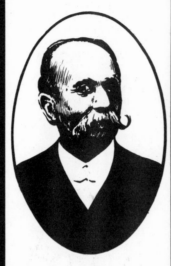

Scottish researcher (Sir) David Ferrier (1843–1928) mapped the motor cortex and found the sensory strip.

Sir William Macewen, a Scot, pioneered successful brain surgery in 1879.

British physiologist Walter Holbrook Gaskell showed in the 1880s that the sympathetic nervous system was not a separate nervous system.

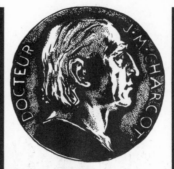

Jean Martin Charcot of Paris (1825–93) helped separate neuroses from psychoses and showed where brain damage causes paralysis and epilepsy.

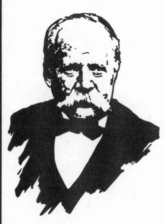

German physiologist Friedrich Goltz in 1892 described loss of all but reflex action in decerebrate dogs.

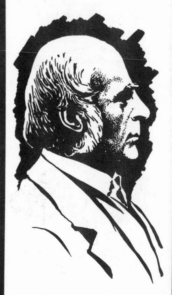

British anthropometrist Sir Francis Galton pioneered the scientific study of the nature of intelligence in 1892.

Heinrick Quincke in 1895 carried out the first lumbar puncture for studying cerebrospinal fluid.

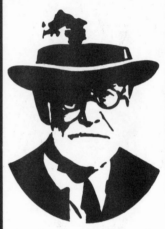

Austrian physician Sigmund Freud pioneered psychoanalysis in the 1890s.

British physiologist John Newport Langley coined the term "autonomic nervous system" in 1898.

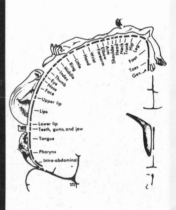

British neurologist John Hughlings Jackson (1835–1911) studied speech defects and muscle spasms respectively due to brain damage and epilepsy. He gave his name to Jacksonian epilepsy, now generally called focal epilepsy. He believed that the brain's main parts represented an evolutionary succession.

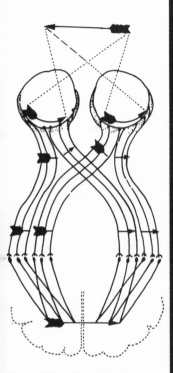

Spanish histologist Santiago Ramón y Cajal (1852–1934) proved that the nervous system consists of a maze of individual cells. He developed a staining technique still in use today.

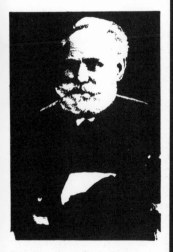

Russian physiologist Ivan Petrovitch Pavlov in the early 1900s discovered conditioned reflexes in dogs.

British researcher Thomas Renton Elliott suggested in 1904 that nerve impulses could be chemically transmitted.

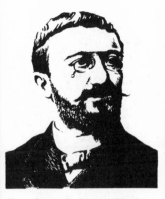

French psychologist Alfred Binet devised tests (1905–11) that made him the "father of modern intelligence testing."

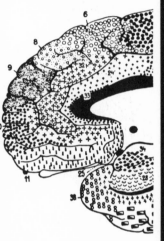

Korbinian Brodmann in 1909 published a "map" of the cerebral cortex which gave numbers to different areas.

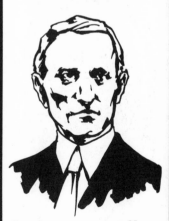

American neurosurgeon Harvey Cushing (1869–1939) invented new brain operations.

British physiologist Keith Lucas (1879–1916) showed the "all or none" response of stimulated neurons.

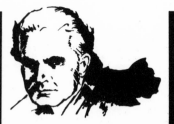

American psychologist John Broadus Watson in 1914 launched behaviorism: a theory claiming that brain activity comprised responses to outside stimuli.

Walter Edward Dandy of Baltimore in 1918 pioneered ventriculography.

Charles Foix of Paris in 1921 located the cause of paralysis agitans in the midbrain's substantia nigra.

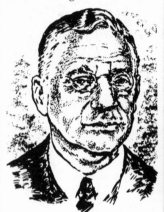

Austrian physiologist Otto Loewi in 1921 discovered effects of a neurotransmitter, acetylcholine.

German researcher Rudolf Magnus in 1926 announced discoveries about how the inner ear regulates balance.

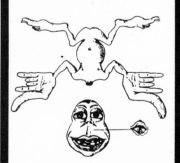

Canadian neurosurgeon Wilder Graves Penfield in and after the late 1920s used microelectrodes to map parts of the human cerebral cortex with differing functions.

©DIAGRAM

Landmarks in Research: 4

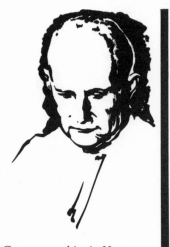

German psychiatrist Hans Berger recorded the first human encephalogram in 1929.

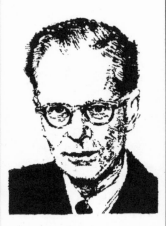

American psychologist Burrhus F. Skinner (inventor of teaching machines) in 1930 described operant conditioning.

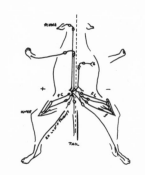

British physiologist Sir Charles Scott Sherrington (1857–1952) made major discoveries of inborn reflexes and showed the central nervous system involves integration of different "levels." He shared a Nobel prize in 1932.

British physiologist Edgar Douglas (Lord) Adrian shared a 1932 Nobel prize for research into the neuron.

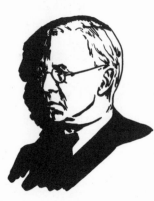

British physiologist Sir Henry Hallett Dale shared a 1936 Nobel prize (with Otto Loewi) for discoveries about chemical transmission of nerve impulses.

J.W. Papez in 1937 suggested the name "limbic system" for the "old mammalian brain" that produces our emotions.

Americans Joseph Erlanger and Herbert Gasser shared a 1944 Nobel prize for studies that involved amplifying the currents in nerves.

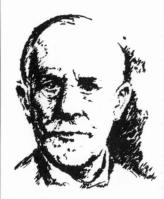

Swiss physiologist Walter Hess shared a 1949 Nobel prize for probing deep-brain function with microelectrodes.

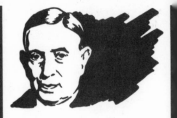

Portuguese neurologist António Caetano de Egas Moniz developed an X-ray technique for studying blood vessels in the brain and in 1949 shared a Nobel prize for pioneering psychosurgery.

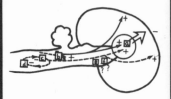

In Illinois in 1949 Giuseppe Moruzzi and Horace Magoun showed that brainstem signals keep the whole brain awake.

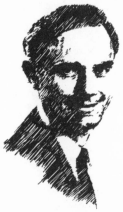

American researcher James Olds in 1953 discovered a pleasure center in the brain.

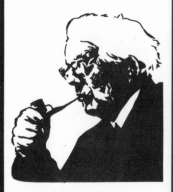

Swiss psychologist Jean Piaget (1896–1980) discovered chronological stages of intellectual development.

American physiologist Vernon Mountcastle in the late 1950s showed that the cortex's nerve cells form a million columns.

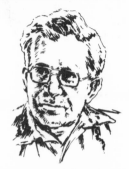

American psycholinguist Noam Chomsky (born 1928) claimed that man's brain is born programed for learning language.

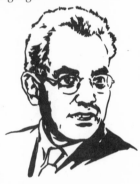

Russian neuropsychologist Alexander R. Luria discovered functional defects produced by local brain damage.

Swedish scientist Holgar Hydén showed in the 1960s that DNA-related changes occur in the brains of rats that have been learning.

British physiologists Alan Lloyd Hodgkin and Andrew Fielding Huxley shared a 1963 Nobel prize for showing (in and after 1952) how ion interchange activates or inhibits nerve impulses.

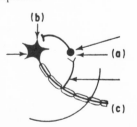

Australian physiologist Sir John Carew Eccles shared a 1963 Nobel prize for research into mechanisms of nerve impulse transmission.

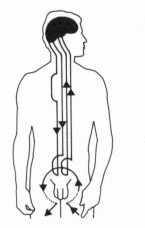

British researchers including Geoffrey Harris in 1965 showed sexuality to be built into the hypothalamus.

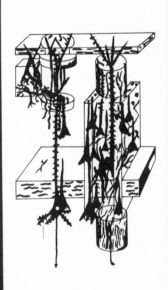

Hungarian neuroanatomist Janos Szentágothai and others in 1967 published a detailed account of the cerebellum.

American psychologist Ulric Neisser in 1967 published *Cognitive Psychology,* a landmark in research understanding thought.

Julius Axelrod (USA), Bernard Katz (Britain) and Svante von Euler (Sweden) shared a 1970 Nobel prize for research into chemicals transmitting nerve impulses.

American neurophysiologist Karl Pribram suggested brain activity resembled holography, a photographic-like process.

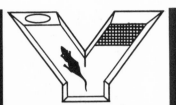

Researching at Houston in the 1970s, Georges Ungar found learning seemed to involve forming peptides in the brain.

In the mid 1970s researchers in the USA and Scotland found brain chemicals that block transmission of pain signals.

By 1980 Swedish and American scientists were transplanting brain tissue in rats.

British neuropsychologist E.T. Rolls in 1980 reported individual neurons deep in the brain, associated with specific types of visual perception.

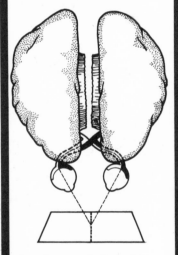

American psychobiologist Roger Sperry shared a 1981 Nobel prize for "split-brain" discoveries begun in 1961.

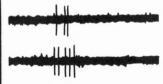

American neurobiologist David Hubel and Swedish colleague Torsten Wiesel shared a 1981 Nobel prize for discoveries (published 1959) of how the brain interprets visual signals.

In Canada in 1982, Martin Benfey and Albert Aguayo showed that damaged brain cells can be persuaded to regrow.

©DIAGRAM

Index

Index

Index